Pain Management: Expanding the Pharmacological Options

Commissioning Editor: Martin Sugden
Development Editor: Jennifer Seward
Production Controller: Debbie Wyer

Pain Management: Expanding the Pharmacological Options

Gary J. McCleane MD FFARCSI DA DipIMC Dip Pain Mang

Consultant in Pain Management
Rampark Pain Centre
Lurgan
Northern Ireland

⟨W⟩WILEY-BLACKWELL

A John Wiley and Sons, Ltd., Publication

This edition first published 2008, © 2008 by Gary J. McCleane

Blackwell Publishing was acquired by John Wiley & Sons in February 2007. Blackwell's publishing program has been merged with Wiley's global Scientific, Technical and Medical business to form Wiley-Blackwell.

Registered office: John Wiley & Sons Ltd, The Atrium, Southern Gate, Chichester, West Sussex, PO19 8SQ, UK

Editorial offices: 9600 Garsington Road, Oxford, OX4 2DQ, UK
The Atrium, Southern Gate, Chichester, West Sussex, PO19 8SQ, UK
111 River Street, Hoboken, NJ 07030-5774, USA

For details of our global editorial offices, for customer services and for information about how to apply for permission to reuse the copyright material in this book please see our website at www.wiley.com/wiley-blackwell

Library of Congress Cataloguing-in-Publication Data
McCleane, Gary.
  Pain management : expanding the pharmacological options / Gary J. McCleane.
    p. ; cm.
  Includes bibliographical references and index.
  ISBN 978-1-4051-7823-5 (alk. paper)
  1. Analgesics. 2. Analgesia. 3. Pain—Treatment. I. Title.
  [DNLM: 1. Pain—drug therapy. 2. Drug Therapy—methods. WL 704 M4776p 2008]
  RM319.M33 2008
  615'.783—dc22

                                                                      2008009436

ISBN: 978-1-4051-7823-5

A catalogue record for this book is available from the British Library.

Set in 9.5/13 pt Meridien by Charon Tec Ltd (A Macmillan Company), Chennai, India
www.charontec.com
Printed in Singapore by Utopia Press Pte Ltd

1 2008

Contents

Foreword

Medicine has made great strides in the 21st century included among which has been the development of new analgesics and novel routes of administration. However, despite these great advances as well as the prospect of future treatment strategies (such as viral vectors and gene therapy), we still cannot guarantee our patients that we can relieve their pain or avoid drug-related side effects. There is still an ongoing need to carefully weigh the risk/benefit ratios of each potential treatment option and it is not difficult to appreciate why treatment strategies associated with few adverse effects may be attractive to patients as well as health care providers. One can see, therefore, that if an analgesic potential is attributed to a medicine that has been available for sometime, previously with a non-pain indication, physicians may have less reluctance to use that medication than an entirely new agent with which there is little patient experience.

The concept of using medication on an "off-label" fashion often causes those who treat patients concern particularly in this era of intense medico-legal scrutiny. Therefore not only are judgments regarding efficacy and risk of adverse effects required when a "novel" pharmacological agent is considered, but also thought needs to be given regarding the confidence with which the practitioner can stand over their decision to prescribe that drug. Fortunately many of the options outlined in this book fall into a "low risk" category in terms of potential side effects and their use for other indications has been extensive. Furthermore, there are bodies of evidence that supports their use and this must give reassurance to those who choose to use them as pain relievers.

The problem of pain and suffering remains an enormous issue in many respects. On one hand there are still too many patients with inadequate analgesia and on the other hand there are too many adverse effects from treatment efforts to achieve adequate analgesia. The use of unconventional pain treatments, unconventional routes of administration, and the use of drugs outside their license indication is an area of increasing interest to many and currently there is no text which covers all of this information in one source. This text will likely appeal to a wide variety of practitioners from many disciplines.

Howard Smith MD

Associate Professor & Director of Pain Management

Albany Medical College

Department of Anesthesiology

Albany, New York, USA

Editor-in-Chief *Journal of Neuropathic Pain & Symptom Palliation*

Editor-in-Chief *Journal of Cancer Pain & Symptom Palliation*

CHAPTER 1

Introduction

One cannot fail to be impressed by the enormous increase in the knowledge of pain mechanisms that have occurred over the last few decades. We now have a much clearer understanding about the processes that convert a noxious stimulus into one that is appreciated as pain. And yet the drugs that would allow us to intervene therapeutically on the basis of this knowledge are often not available and indeed seem some way off. Granted there is a steady stream of products released by the pharmaceutical industry, but when examined in more detail these are often old compounds reformulated or imitations of currently available drugs.

When one thinks of "conventional" pain treatment, one thinks of opioids which have been used historically for millennia, nonsteroidal anti-inflammatories and local anesthetics which have their genesis over one hundred years ago and even the tricyclic antidepressants which are now over 40 years old. It is true, however, that while the basic pain-relieving drugs that are currently used could be recognized by practitioners from a previous generation, our thoughts about how they are used have been, and keep, changing. There is, for example, less reluctance to use strong opioids for chronic pain, and tricyclic antidepressants and anti-epileptic are often initiated by General Practitioners, which were previously used in the realm of specialist practice. In addition, patient expectation has changed from a stoical acceptance of pain to an expectation that pain is not acceptable and that there must be a remedy for it. With an aging population and patients recovering from previously irrecoverable illness, but with pain sequelae, the need for effective pain treatment has never been greater and yet the fundamental question remains as to whether we have the ability to effectively treat all pain. It is beyond contention that the answer to that question is no. Even if currently available drugs were effective in all cases, which they are not, the side effects produced by these drugs are not infrequently unacceptable to the patient. And

Pain Management: Expanding the Pharmacological Options, Gary J. McCleane. © 2008 Blackwell Publishing, ISBN: 978-1-4051-7823-5.

these are only the immediate and obvious side effects of those preparations. The majority of pain drug studies examine the effect and side effect profiles of these medications over just a few weeks. We have few long-term studies of the effects of sustained use of opioids, anti-epileptics, or other drugs used in pain management.

If one went further and proposed that only drugs with a licensed indication could be considered for the treatment of pain in a particular condition then the choice, and indeed chances, of successful treatment are further reduced. The issue of drug use outside its specific licence is one which exorcizes practitioners and leaves them feeling vulnerable if they use a medication for the very best of reasons but when its use is complicated by adverse effect.

On the other hand, it would be unrealistic to expect the pharmaceutical industry to invest the many millions needed to obtain a product licence unless they can recoup their initial investment. This is only possible if they own the Intellectual Property rights to that preparation, or combination of preparations, and can therefore gain patent protection for their developments. One is therefore left with a relatively small number of pharmacological entities with proven analgesic effect which possess an indication for use in a particular pain condition. Everyday practice confirms that choice from such a small group is not always rewarded with pain relief. So what does one do? Explain to the patients that there are no further alternatives or try other low-risk pharmacological strategies that may bring relief?

It is staggering to see the number of scientific papers published month in, month out, on the genesis, transmission, control, and non-clinical treatment of pain. Although not all this work sheds new light on our understanding, the knowledge presented pushes us closer to the goal of complete understanding. This wisdom is only of real use if it helps us to reduce suffering. In some cases it will indicate how an entirely new pharmacological approach can be taken to pain treatment. In other, and probably more, cases it indicates receptors and pathways which we can interact with currently available medication. Such opportunities may allow us to interfere with pain transmission and regulation with drugs which we are familiar with, but for whom there is an entirely different indication. We often have vast experience in using these drugs for other non-pain indications and this means that their use may be inside the "comfort zone" of many more practitioners. It is less likely that negative information will emerge about long-term use since their pre-pain use will have already been long term.

Some will argue that the use of such "unconventional" treatments represent the use of medication for pain in which there is no evidence base. This is rarely the case. Indeed, for many of the treatments to be described, a substantial body of preclinical evidence rationalizes their use and this evidence is confirmed by human clinical trials. Granted there may be fewer human pain trials on these currently unlicensed drugs but this is hardly surprising as these studies are usually unfunded by the pharmaceutical industry (in direct contrast to those studies on licensed preparations) and so the ability of investigators to assess the pain-relieving effects of these medications is lessened. It cannot be contended that the presence of a pain licence for a particular medication confirms or even suggests that it is the best agent for that type of pain. Rather it tells us that the company who hold the licence have assessed that the financial investment needed to obtain a licence will be offset by sufficient profit from its sale.

Even if evidence of analgesic effect were weaker for some of the medications to be discussed, absence of evidence of effect may only indicate that appropriate studies have not yet been undertaken to prove the effect. To ignore these older drugs which have current non-pain indications would be to ignore the results of basic science investigation that now suggest that they may have useful pain-relieving properties. Given that these older agents often have modes of action which are entirely different to that of currently licensed pain drugs, the use of these older drugs gives new opportunity for pain relief, as previously inaccessible receptors or pathways can be influenced by their use. Is there more logic in trying to assault the same receptor or pathway repeatedly with currently available medication and the copycat forms of it, or to try to access previously inaccessible receptors or pathways? Surely the logic is that faced with therapeutic failure with one type of agent the use of another agent with a different mode of action entirely would be more appropriate.

As anybody dealing with patients will know, it is not unusual to be faced with a patient who fails to respond to the normal pain relief provided, cannot take it because of side effects, or cannot use it because of contraindications. One thinks of the patient with renal impairment in whom the use of non-steroidal anti-inflammatories would be contraindicated and yet has a pain in which tissue inflammation is prominent or the patient with postherpetic neuralgia who cannot afford sleepiness and cognitive impairment associated with tricyclic antidepressant or anti-epileptic use. What do you then do? Or think of the patient with a terminal illness in whom the last days of life risk being ruined by pain, or by the side effects of currently accepted pain medication. Would it not be better if there was a simple, low-risk treatment that would give pain relief without the side effects which, for example, are found with opioid use? It is to suggest options for scenarios such as these that this book exists. The alternatives suggested are not guaranteed to work and are not guaranteed to be free of side effects, but then neither is more conventional treatment. No one analgesic option is universally effective or acceptable for the patient. With a wider range of options whose use is based on logic, then the chances of therapeutic success must be increased.

The focus of this book, therefore, is on widening the available choice of drugs which the practitioner has to choose from when trying to optimalize pain management for the patient should they have acute pain, chronic pain, or the pain associated with a terminal illness. The intention is that by having a wider armamentarium the practitioner can tailor the patient's treatment to provide that patient with the most effective pain treatment with the fewest number of side effects resulting from treatment. By reducing the number of drugs to just those with the licensed indication, the chances of success must be significantly reduced. Furthermore, the evidence base which supports the use of these seemingly novel alternatives will be indicated so that the reader can either accept that there is evidence or explore that evidence to see if it backs up the claims made for these drugs. The ethos of the book is intended to be that the choice of pain-relieving medication should be guided by the published scientific evidence and not by what the drug industry feels able to invest in. There is a difference between these philosophies. By at least considering the former there must be some chance that we can enhance the pain relief provided to the patient.

CHAPTER 2

Conventional Pain Treatment

In the past pain treatment revolved around the use of a small number of drugs. Mild pain was treated with paracetamol/acetaminophen with or without a non-steroidal anti-inflammatory (NSAID), whereas pain of a more severe nature was treated with codeine-based preparations, often in combination with paracetamol/acetaminophen. When postoperative pain was being managed, strong opioids were and are still utilized.

Perhaps one of the most major advances in recent decades has not been the advent of new analgesic agents, but rather an understanding that not all pain is the same with the implication that not all pain treatment can be standardized. We now appreciate that postoperative pain differs from the pain experienced with chronic conditions such as osteoarthritis (OA) while neuropathic pain differs yet again. The management of pain in each of these scenarios is now reasonably standardized and often governed by recommendations from professional organizations, colleges, and other interested parties. A greater proportion of the drugs utilized have a specific indication for the use to which they are put. However, some do not, and yet, because of a sufficient body of trial evidence and clinical experience are widely accepted and used. For example, the tricyclic antidepressants (TCAs) are universally accepted to have a pain-reducing effect in a variety of neuropathic pain conditions and in patients with fibromyalgia, are extensively used in these conditions and yet do not have a licensed indication for pain in these conditions. The whole issue of "off-label" use will be examined in more depth in the next chapter.

An up-to-date selection of guidelines can be accessed at the website of the *National Guideline Clearinghouse*, a US-based site but which contains guidelines from around the world. It can be found at: www.guideline.gov.

There is clearly much merit in benefiting from the considered opinions of consensus panels that formulate these guidelines. However, four issues arise when the guidelines are consulted:

1 They contain the first-line treatment options rather than the options utilized in specialist practice.

Pain Management: Expanding the Pharmacological Options, Gary J. McCleane. © 2008
Blackwell Publishing, ISBN: 978-1-4051-7823-5.

2 The therapeutic options presented, which include labeled and off-labeled drug use, are included because of the weight of evidence of their pain-relieving effects. However, that does not necessarily mean that these are the best options, merely that they have been more rigorously investigated. We lack good studies of comparative effect.

3 The process of drug discovery, investigation, release, and the interval between release and acceptance by practitioners and ultimately by the consensus panels that formulate guidelines imposes a time delay that may make the subsequent guideline dated.

4 The guidelines concentrate on specific diseases and causes of pain such as postherpetic neuralgia and OA. For many conditions no guidelines exist.

Neuropathic pain

Pain arising from injury or irritation of neural tissue may result in neuropathic pain. This pain has characteristic features which distinguish it from pain arising from noxious stimulation of other non-neural structures.

Accepted treatment for neuropathic pain involves the use of three distinct classes of medication:

1 Opioids

2 Antidepressants – Tricyclic antidepressants (TCAs) and serotonin norepinephrine reuptake inhibitors (SNRIs)

3 Antiepileptic drugs (AEDs)

While other types of medication are used, these three groups form the mainstay of treatment.

There is clear advantage on forming treatment around these groups. However, few would contend that therapeutic success is guaranteed when these types of drugs are used either because they prove ineffective or because their use is complicated by unacceptable side effects.

The causes of neuropathic pain are legion: while postherpetic neuralgia and painful diabetic neuropathy are perhaps the most well known, an extensive list of other types could easily be formulated. And yet, no TCA has a specific indication or licence for use in neuropathic pain but their use in these conditions is extensive. In the USA, two AEDs have neuropathic pain-related indications. These are gabapentin which has an indication for postherpetic neuralgia and pregabalin which has an indication for postherpetic neuralgia and painful diabetic neuropathy. No AED has an indication for ilioinguinal neuritis, intercostal neuritis or genitofemoral neuralgia, for example.

It can clearly be seen, therefore, that there would be severe limitations in our ability to provide effective treatment if we were to utilize medication only according to its labeled use.

Two current guidelines advise on the management of neuropathic pain in general. In the first of these, Dworkin and colleagues (2003) suggest:

First line-medications. The efficacy of gabapentin, the 5% lidocaine patch, opioid analgesics, tramadol hydrochloride, and tricyclic antidepressants has been consistently demonstrated in multiple randomized trials.

Second line-medications. When patients do not have a satisfactory response to treatment with the five first-line medications alone or in combination, several medications can be considered second-line. The list of second-line medications include:

- lamotrigine
- carbamazepine
- bupropion
- citalopram
- paroxetine
- venlafaxine.

Beyond second-line medications: Other medications sometimes used for the treatment of patients with neuropathic pain include capsaicin, clonidine, dextromethorphan, and mexiletine.

In a more recent guideline representing the views of the *Canadian Pain Society* (2007) the suggestions are:

First-line treatments
- Tricyclic antidepressants
- Gabapentin & pregabalin

Second-line treatments
- Serotonin noradrenaline reuptake inhibitors.
- Topical lidocaine

Third-line treatments
- Tramadol
- Controlled release opioids

Fourth-line treatments
- Cannabinoids
- Methadone
- Lamotrigine
- Topiramate
- Valproic acid.

A guideline specific to postherpetic neuralgia has been formulated by the *American Academy of Neurology* (2004). Its major recommendations are:

1 Tricyclic antidepressants, gabapentin, pregabalin, opioids, and topical lidocaine patches are effective and should be used in the treatment of postherpetic neuralgia.

2 Aspirin in cream is possibly effective in the relief of pain in patients with postherpetic neuralgia, but the magnitude of benefit is low, as is seen with capsaicin.

3 In countries where preservative-free intrathecal methylprednisolone is available, it may be considered in the treatment of postherpetic neuralgia.

4 Acupuncture, benzydamine cream, dextromethorphan, indomethacin, epidural methylprednisolone, epidural morphine sulphate, iontophoresis of vincristine, lorazepam, vitamin E, and zimelidine are not of benefit.

5 The effectiveness of carbamazepine, nicardipine, biperiden, chlorprothixene, ketamine, helium, neon laser irradiation, intralesional triamcinolone, cryocautery, topical piroxicam, extract of Ganoderma lucidum, dorsal root entry zone lesions, and stellate ganglion block are unproven in the treatment of postherpetic neuralgia.

The only other neuropathic pain condition that currently has a guideline is complex regional pain syndrome. This guideline has been produced by the *Reflex Sympathetic Dystrophy Association* (2006). It suggests:

- Mild to moderate pain: Simple analgesics and/or blocks
- Excruciating, intractable pain: Opioids and/or blocks
- Inflammation/swelling and edema: Steroids, systemic or targeted or NSAIDs; immunomodulators
- Depression, anxiety, insomnia: Sedative, analgesic antidepressant/anxiolytics
- Significant allodynia/hyperalgesia: Anticonvulsants and/or other sodium channel blockers and or N-methyl-D-aspartate receptor antagonists

A single drug rather than disease guideline concentrates on the use of AEDs in pain management. It comes from the *Washington State Department of Labor and Industries*. It gives guidance into which AEDs can be used by physicians and attract reimbursement from the department. It states:

Currently, there is a lack of evidence to demonstrate that AEDs significantly reduce the level of acute pain, myofascial pain, low back pain, or other sources of somatic pain. The evidence of efficacy and safety on AEDs in the treatment of neuropathic pain varies and depends on the specific agent in this drug class.

Gabapentin, along with older antiepileptic drugs, may be used as a first-line therapy in the treatment of chronic neuropathic pain. Because evidence of efficacy with lamotrigine has been inconsistent and there is no evidence of efficacy and safety for levetiracetam, oxcarbazepine, tiagabine, topiramate, and zonisamide, these drugs will not routinely be covered by the department for the treatment of neuropathic pain.

If one takes the messages from these guidelines and extends them into clinical practice there is still a very real chance that pain relief will not be apparent. One is again left with the dilemma of whether to explain to the patient that no other therapeutic intervention is available for them or to try drugs not considered "conventional" and yet which are suggested by a careful reading of the literature. It is around this latter concept that this book is formed.

Postoperative pain

The management of postoperative pain is perhaps the most regimented of all the types of pain that we treat. At the basis of all postoperative pain treatment is the use of a small number of therapeutic classes of drugs. Local anesthetics, NSAIDs, acetaminophen/paracetamol, and opioids are the mainstays of treatment. Sophisticated postoperative pain management involves the logical use of these drugs delivered by differing varying routes:

Acetaminophen/paracetamol
- Rectal
- Oral
- Intravenous

Local anesthetics
- Skin infiltration
- Nerve blocks
- Epidural
- Intrathecal

Opioids
- Rectal
- Oral
- Transdermal
- Intravenous
- Intramuscular
- Epidural
- Intrathecal

Non-steroidal anti-inflammatory drugs
- Rectal
- Oral
- Intramuscular
- Intravenous

Combination therapy is the cornerstone of postoperative pain management. Problems arise when it is not possible to use one of the constituents of our combinations. For example, NSAIDs may have to be withheld in the patient with severe dyspepsia, previous NSAID allergy, those on anticoagulants, or when there is significant renal impairment. While the worst excesses of pain can be reduced or removed by regional anesthetic techniques, when these are discontinued acetaminophen/paracetamol and opioid combinations may not be sufficient to provide good quality relief.

The primacy of multimodal postoperative pain management is emphasized by the *American Society of Anesthesiologists* Task Force on Acute Pain Management (2004):

> Whenever possible, anesthesiologists should employ multimodal pain management therapy. Unless contraindicated, all patients should receive an around-the-clock regimen of non-steroidal anti-inflammatory drugs (NSAIDs), cyclo-oxygenase-2 inhibitors (COXIBs), or acetaminophen. In addition, regional blockade with local anesthetics should be considered. Dosing regimens should be administered to optimize efficacy while minimizing the risk of adverse events. The choice of medication, dose, route, and duration of therapy should be individualized.

Musculoskeletal pain

Relatively few general guidelines exist for musculoskeletal pain management. As with neuropathic pain, they tend to concentrate on one particular type and source of pain. One example is a guideline formulated by the *American Academy of Orthopedic Surgeons* (2003). In terms of pharmacological therapy they suggest a trial of an analgesic, non-steroidal anti-inflammatory or acetaminophen. If this fails a further option is that of joint aspiration and injection of cortisone, although they rate the strength of evidence for this recommendation as "little or no systematic empirical evidence." They go on to state that the role of "chondroprotective" agents such as glucosamine and chondroitin sulfate in the treatment of OA is not yet clear.

A European perspective is given by the *European League Against Rheumatism* (EULAR) guidelines for the management of OA of the hip (2005). Their suggestions for the pharmacological treatment of OA hip are:

- Paracetamol/acetaminophen as the oral analgesic of first choice for mild to moderate pain.
- NSAIDs at the lowest effective dose for those who fail to respond satisfactorily to paracetamol/acetaminophen.
- Opioids with or without paracetamol/acetaminophen as alternatives to NSAIDs when they are ineffective, poorly tolerated or contraindicated.
- Glucosamine, chondroitin, diacerhein, avocado soybean, and hyaluronic acid may be used although their effects are not well established.
- Intra-articular steroid injections during a flare up when NSAIDs or analgesics are ineffective.

In a further EULAR guideline (2007), this time for the management of hand OA, of the 17 treatment modalities considered, only 6 were supported by research evidence. These were education plus exercise, NSAIDs, COX-2 inhibitors, topical NSAIDs, topical capsaicin, and chondroitin sulfate.

Cancer pain

Perhaps in no other field of pain management is a systematic approach more important than in the field of cancer pain management. Provision of analgesia represents only one strand of management with thought needing to be given to the full panoply of physical and emotional aspects of the individual patient's condition. One of the revolutions in pain management was the institution of the *World Health Organization* analgesic ladder. This concentrated attention on a graded approach to provision of pain relief and emphasized the need to institute strong opioid therapy when pain becomes resistant to simpler analgesic options.

A wide variety of treatment guidelines now exist for cancer pain management and that of the *American Pain Society* (2005) suggests in terms of pharmacological management:

- Provide cancer patients with a prescription for an analgesic medication (e.g., hydrocodone and acetaminophen, oxycodone with acetaminophen) and instruct patients to have the prescription filled, to take the medication if unexpected pain occurs, and to call their healthcare provider for an appointment to evaluate the pain problem.
- Base the initial treatment of cancer pain on the severity of the pain the patient reports.
- Begin a bowel regimen to prevent constipation when the patient is started on an opioid analgesic.
- Administer a long-acting opioid on an around-the-clock basis, along with an immediate-release opioid to be used on an as-needed basis, for breakthrough pain once the patient's pain intensity and dose are stabilized.
- Do not use meperidine in the management of chronic cancer pain.
- Adjust opioid doses for each patient to achieve pain relief with an acceptable level of side effects.
- Avoid intramuscular administration because it is painful and absorption is not reliable.
- Use optimally titrated doses of opioids and maximal safe and tolerable doses of co-analgesics through other routes of administration before considering spinal analgesics.
- Monitor for and prophylactically treat opioid-induced side effects.
- Titrate naloxone, when in the rare instances it is indicated for the reversal of opioid-induced respiratory depression, by giving incremental doses that improve respiratory function but do not reverse analgesia.
- Provide patients and family caregivers with accurate and understandable information about effective cancer pain management, the use of analgesic medications, other methods of pain control, and how to communicate effectively with clinicians about unrelieved cancer pain.

- Provide patients with a written pain management plan.
- Use cognitive and behavioral strategies as part of a multimodal approach to cancer pain management, not as a replacement for analgesic medication.

Fibromyalgia

Those with an interest in rheumatological conditions will know all too well the significant burden of patients with pain associated with fibromyalgia.

The American Pain Society suggest in their *Clinical Practice Guideline* of 2005 the following rules when treating fibromyalgia syndrome (FMS) pharmacologically while pointing out that treatment should also be non-pharmacological as well:

1 For initial treatment of FMS prescribe a TCA for sleep.
2 Use selective serotonin reuptake inhibitors (SSRIs) alone, or in combination with tricyclics, for pain relief.
3 Do not use NSAIDs as the primary pain medication for people with FMS. There is no evidence that NSAIDs are effective when used alone to treat FMS patients.
4 Use tramadol for pain relief in patients with FMS.
5 Use opioids for management of FMS pain only after all other pharmacologic and non-pharmacologic therapies have been exhausted.
6 Use sleep and anti-anxiety medications if sleep disturbances such as restless leg syndrome are prominent.
7 Do not use corticosteroids in the treatment of FMS unless there is concurrent joint, bursa, or tendon inflammation.

A different guideline for the management of FMS has been formulated by Goldenberg and colleagues (2004). They classify drug treatment into those according to the evidence of efficacy:

Strong evidence for efficacy
- Amitriptyline
- Cyclobenzaprine

Modest evidence for efficacy
- Tramadol
- Serotonin reuptake inhibitors (SSRIs)
- Dual-reuptake inhibitors (SNRIs)
- Pregabalin

Weak evidence for efficacy
- Growth hormone
- 5-hydroxytryptamine
- Tropisetron
- *S*-adenosyl-methionine

No evidence for efficacy
- Opioids
- Corticosteroids

- NSAIDs
- Benzodiazepine and non-benzodiazepine hypnotics
- Melatonin
- Calcitonin
- Thyroid hormone
- Guaifenesin
- Dehydroepiandrosterone
- Magnesium

Conclusions

There is no doubt that the guidelines that cover a relatively small number of the conditions that cause pain offer a sound basis for pain treatment and their message can be extended to many other pain conditions. However, those involved in patient treatment will know that the therapeutic modalities suggested in these guidelines are not universally effective in all patients, nor are they universally well tolerated. In this age of resource shortage, the failure to respond to guideline treatment can lead to a discharge from the care of the treating physician with the message being conveyed that all has been tried and nothing more can be done. It could be argued that such a discharge from care equates to a discharge of responsibility. From a humanitarian perspective this is not acceptable. In some fields such as in the care of the dying patient the discharge approach would be entirely unacceptable. And yet what does one do? It is suggested that one approach may be to be mindful of the available pain literature and use the scientific validation contained in it to try other pharmacological strategies that often come with a real chance of providing pain relief along with a low chance of adverse effects.

Bibliography

American Academy of Orthopedic Surgeons. AAOS clinical practice guideline on osteoarthritis of the knee. *American Academy of Orthopedic Surgeons*. Rosemont, Illinois, 2003, p. 17.

American Society of Anesthesiologists Task Force on Acute Pain Management. Practice guidelines for acute pain management in the postoperative setting: an updated report by the American Society of Anesthesiologists Task Force on Acute Pain Management. *Anesthesiology* 2004; 100: 1573–81.

Burckhardt CS, Goldenberg D, Crofford L et al. Guideline for the management of fibromyalgia syndrome pain in adults and children. *American Pain Society*. Glenview, Illinois, 2005, p. 109 (Clinical Practice Guideline No. 4).

Dubinsky RM, Kabbani H, El-Chami Z et al. Practice parameter: treatment of postherpetic neuralgia: an evidence-based report of the Quality Standards Subcommittee of the American Academy of Neurology. *Neurology* 2004; 63: 959–65.

Dworkin RH, Backonja M, Rowbotham MC et al. Advances in neuropathic pain: diagnosis, mechanisms, and treatment recommendations. *Arch Neurol* 2003; 60: 1524–34.

European League Against Rheumatism. EULAR evidence based recommendations for the management of hip osteoarthritis. *Ann Rheum Dis* 2007; 64: 669–81.

Goldenberg DL, Burckhardt C, Crofford L. Management of fibromyalgia syndrome. *JAMA* 2004; 292: 2388–95.

Miaskowski C, Cleary J, Burney R et al. Guideline for the management of cancer pain in adults and children. *American Pain Society.* Glenview, Illinois 2005; p. 166.

Moulin DE, Clark AJ, Gilron I et al. Pharmacological management of chronic neuropathic pain – consensus statement and guidelines from the Canadian Pain Society. *Pain Res Manage* 2007; 12: 13–21.

Reflex Sympathetic Dystrophy Syndrome Association (RSDSA). Complex regional pain syndrome: treatment guidelines. Reflex Sympathetic Dystrophy Syndrome Association, Milford, Connecticut, 2006, p. 67.

Washington State Department of Labor and Industries. Antiepileptic drugs guideline for chronic pain. *Provider Bull* 2005; 05–10: 1–3.

Zhang W, Doherty M, Leeb BF et al. EULAR evidence based recommendations for the management of hand osteoarthritis: report of a Task Force of the EULAR Standing Committee for International Clinical Studies Including Therapeutics (ESCISIT). *Ann Rheum Dis* 2007; 66: 377–88.

CHAPTER 3

Using Drugs Outside Their Licensed Indication

As can be seen in the preceding chapter, useful guidance on the management of a wide variety of pain conditions is provided by published guidelines. These guidelines represent the considered views of consensus panels and are based on the available published evidence. Although there is much merit in their use, significant and important aspects of pain control are not contained within them.

The medications recommended are often, but not always, licensed by the regulatory authorities for their use in these conditions. When "conventional" therapies fail to provide relief, less conventional treatments can be recommended, and it is much more common in these circumstances for the suggested drugs not to have a specific licence for use in that condition. When these options are suggested, it is not unusual for other practitioners to express concern about their unlicensed, off-label use. In reality, even these practitioners often prescribe medication off-label. For example, the use of a tricyclic antidepressant (TCA) for its sleep-enhancing and analgesic effect is usual in patients who receive a diagnosis of fibromyalgia, and yet no TCA has a licence for use in patients with fibromyalgia.

Drug licensing and approval

The system of drug licensing and approval differs depending on the country involved. In the UK, for example, this process is regulated by the Medicines and Healthcare products Regulatory Agency (MHRA), whereas in the USA this function is fulfilled by the Food and Drug Administration (FDA).

United Kingdom

A comprehensive medicines regulatory system was introduced in the UK in 1971 as set out in the Medicines Act of that year. This system

Pain Management: Expanding the Pharmacological Options, Gary J. McCleane. © 2008
Blackwell Publishing, ISBN: 978-1-4051-7823-5.

introduced licensing affecting the manufacture, sale, supply, and importation of medicinal products into the UK. During subsequent years the UK and other member states of the European Union (EU) contributed to the development and updating of EU Directives in this area. European Union legislation now takes precedence over the UK Medicines Act.

It is the responsibility of the MHRA and its advisory bodies to ensure the balance between the safety and effectiveness of a medicine. To this end all applications for approval are assessed by the experts of the MHRA. This process is followed up by a system of inspecting and testing which continues throughout the lifetime of the medicine. Before a medicine is sold in the UK a licence called a "marketing authorization" (formerly called a "product licence") must be sought from the MHRA. New products which are still under development also need a licence before they can be tested on human subjects. This "clinical trial authorization" is also obtained by application through the MHRA.

The criteria for a marketing authorization are based on the following three criteria only:
• The safety of the medicine
• The quality of the medicine
• The efficacy of the medicine

All the medications to be discussed in forthcoming chapters do not have a "marketing authorization" in UK terms, or are "off-label" in US terms for the uses to be described. However, they do have "marketing authorization" for other non-pain indications and hence the safety and quality criteria have been assessed to the satisfaction of the regulatory authorities.

United States of America

The FDA is a federal agency within the Department of Health and Human Services with the responsibility to regulate and evaluate products for human and animal use that are applied to or taken within the body. As in the UK, they ensure that:
• Products should be labeled with the ingredients
• The product should be safe
• The product should be effective

To that end the FDA is based around the scientific principles that:
1 they perform risk analysis and assessment to monitor studies on unapproved products,
2 they evaluate claims about products for safety and efficacy and grant marketing licences, and
3 they monitor products after approval for continued risk assessment.

When there is sufficient data to consider a product safe and effective for a particular use, the information is summarized and assembled into a "New Drug Application." A multidisciplinary team of FDA scientists conduct a review and determine whether the proposed claim can be granted a marketing licence based on the potential risks and benefits. Importantly, it is not a new drug that is approved or not approved but rather the claim about the new drug. Approval may not be granted if:

– there is insufficient evidence to support the claim,
– the risks are considered unacceptable,
– the FDA and the sponsor cannot come to agreement about the scope or wording of the claim.

Any approved product may be used by a licensed practitioner for uses other than those stated in the product label. Off-label use is not illegal, but means that the data to support that use have not been independently reviewed by the FDA.

Regulation of Medical Practitioners

In the UK, the practice of medicine is regulated by the General Medical Council. If an individual doctor's practice strays outside what is deemed acceptable, then they leave themselves open to a charge of professional misconduct which the General Medical Council may deem to be of a degree that would warrant restrictions on that practitioner's practice or even for them to withdraw from that individual their licence to practice.

In the context of the use of unlicensed medication the General Medical Council sets out its view in its booklet *Good Medical Practice* (2001):

Prescribing Medicines for use outside the terms of their licence (off-label)

19. You may prescribe medicines for purposes for which they are not licensed.
20. When prescribing a medicine for use outside the terms of its licence you must:
    a. Be satisfied that it would better serve the patient's needs than an appropriately licensed alternative.
    b. Be satisfied that there is a sufficient evidence base and / or experience of using the medicine to demonstrate its safety and efficacy. The manufacturer's information may be of limited help in which case the necessary information must be sought from other sources.
    c. Take responsibility for prescribing the medicine and for overseeing the patient's care, monitoring and any follow up treatment, or arrange for another doctor to do so.
    d. Make a clear, accurate and legible record of all medicines prescribed and, where you are not following common practice, your reasons for prescribing the medicine.

The General Medical Council goes on to give guidance about what information should be provided to patients about the medication they take:

Information for patients about the licence for their medicines

21. You must give patients, or those authorising treatment on their behalf, sufficient information about the proposed course of treatment, including any known serious or common side effects or adverse reactions.

22. Some medicines are routinely used outside the scope of their licence, for example in treating children. Where current practice supports the use of a medicine in this way it may not be necessary to draw attention to the licence when seeking consent. However, it is good practice to give as much information as patients, or those authorising treatment on their behalf, require or which they may see as significant. Where patients, or their carers express concern you should explain, in broad terms, the reasons why medicines are not licensed for their proposed use. Such explanations may be supported by written information.

23. However, you must explain the reasons for prescribing a medicine that is unlicensed or being outside the scope of its licence where there is little research or other evidence of current practice to support its use, or the use of the medicine is innovative.

In the US, the American Medical Association state in their opinion *E-8.06 Prescribing and dispensing drugs and devices* (2002):

Physicians should prescribe drugs, devices, and other treatments based solely upon medical considerations and patient need and reasonable expectations of the effectiveness of the drug, device or other treatment for the particular patient.

The American Medical Association have also provided testimony to the US Senate Committee on Health, Education, Labor, and Pensions in 2005 that they recommend the "preservation of off-label prescribing" and further that "the FDA should ensure that physicians' ability to prescribe drugs off-label not be impeded."

Pain-relieving drugs

In the UK, the drugs listed in Table 3.1 hold the noted marketing authorizations.

Quite clearly, if one were to restrict the choice of pain-relieving drug to only those with a licence for use in that particular condition, then that choice would be limited or in certain circumstances non-existent.

In the USA, similar narrow indications exist for many of the drugs noted above. For example, the label for gabapentin is for postherpetic neuralgia, that for pregabalin is for postherpetic neuralgia and painful diabetic neuropathy, while that for topical lidocaine is also for postherpetic neuralgia.

Table 3.1 Drugs and their marketing authorization in the UK.

Drug class	Drug	Marketing authorization
Simple analgesic	Paracetamol	Mild to moderate pain
Opioids	Buprenorphine	Moderate to severe pain
		Postoperative pain
	Codeine	Mild to moderate pain
	Dihydrocodeine	Moderate to severe pain
	Dipipanone	Moderate to severe pain
	Fentanyl	Breakthrough pain
		Chronic intractable pain
	Hydromorphone	Severe pain in cancer
	Meptazinol	Moderate to severe pain
		Postoperative and obstetric pain
		Perioperative pain
		Pain and renal colic
	Methadone	Severe pain
	Nefopam	Moderate pain
	Oxycodone	Moderate to severe pain in patients with cancer
		Postoperative pain
		Severe pain
	Papaveretum	Postoperative analgesia
		Severe chronic pain
	Pentazocine	Moderate to severe pain
	Pethidine	Moderate to severe pain
		Obstetric analgesia
		Perioperative analgesia
	Tramadol	Moderate to severe pain
Antidepressants	Duloxetine	Painful diabetic neuropathy
Antiepileptic drugs	Carbamazepine	Trigeminal neuralgia
	Gabapentin	Neuropathic pain
	Pregabalin	Peripheral neuropathic pain
	Phenytoin	Trigeminal neuralgia
Muscle relaxants	Baclofen	Chronic severe spasticity resulting from disorders such as multiple sclerosis (MS)
	Botulinum B toxin	Spasmodic torticollis
	Carisoprodol	Short-term relief of muscle spasm
	Dantrolene	Chronic severe spasticity
	Diazepam	Muscle spasm of varied etiology
	Methocarbamol	Short-term relief of muscle spasm
	Tizanadine	Spasticity associated with MS or spinal injury or disease
Non-steroidal anti-inflammatory drugs	Aceclofenac	Pain in rheumatoid and osteoarthritis
	Celecoxib	
	Etoricoxib	
	Nabumetone	

(Continued)

Table 3.1 (Continued)

Drug class	Drug	Marketing authorization
	Diflunisal	Pain in rheumatoid arthritis and other musculoskeletal conditions
	Fenbrufen	
	Indomethacin	
	Naproxen	
	Piroxicam	
	Sulindac	
	Tenoxicam	
	Tiaprofenic acid	
	Acemetacin	Pain in rheumatic disease and other musculoskeletal disorders
	Diclofenac	Postoperative pain
	Ibuprofen	Pain in rheumatic disease and other musculoskeletal disorders
	Flurbiprofen	Mild to moderate pain Postoperative pain
	Dexibuprofen	Pain in osteoarthritis and other musculoskeletal disorders; Mild to moderate pain
	Dexketoprofen	Short-term treatment of mild to moderate pain
	Fenprofen	Pain in rheumatoid arthritis and other musculoskeletal disorders; Mild to moderate pain
	Ketoprofen	Pain in rheumatoid arthritis and other musculoskeletal disorders; Pain after orthopedic surgery
	Lumiracoxib	Pain in osteoarthritis; Moderate to severe pain associated with orthopedic and dental surgery
	Mefanamic acid	Mild to moderate pain in rheumatoid arthritis, osteoarthritis, and related conditions; Postoperative analgesia; Exacerbation of osteoarthritis (short term)
Others	Local corticosteroids	Injection for local inflammation of joints and soft tissues
	Topical Lidocaine	Postherpetic neuralgia
	Capsaicin	Postherpetic neuralgia; Osteoarthritis

It is therefore suggested that the presence of a "marketing authoriza-tion" or approved indication for an individual drug merely confirms the physical quality of that drug and that the evidence presented to the regulatory authority has been sufficient to reassure them of the safety and efficacy of the drug for that indication. Conversely, the absence of a "marketing authorization" or approved indication suggests either that the regulatory authorities are not satisfied with the quality of the drug or that the evidence of safety or effectiveness of that drug in that indication is inconclusive or that the evidence has not been submitted to them.

As the processes involved in submission to the regulatory authorities are complex and the burden of proof that a drug is safe and effective is relatively high, there is a significant cost associated with the accumulation of evidence and submission. Therefore submissions are undertaken by pharmaceutical companies who perceive their investment in submission can be offset by the profit made from subsequent sale of the drug. They will not be able to recoup their investment in submission unless they have the exclusivity of sale of that drug offered by ownership of the intellectual property rights and hence patent for that drug. Unfortunately this means that if a new pain-relieving effect is established with a drug that is already available for another indication, then there is unlikely to be patent protection available for any company to take on a pain submission to the authorities. This results in having a significant number of drugs available which have a strong pain-relieving effect but which will never be in possession of regulatory approval for a pain indication. It is on these drugs that the latter chapters of this book concentrate. That said, since these drugs have been previously authorized for other non-pain indications, the authorities have already been satisfied as to their quality and safety. It is only on the matter of efficacy in particular conditions that the evidence has not been presented.

With the options to be outlined later, their use is suggested by a strong body of preclinical and clinical evidence. Therefore the stipulation of the like of the General Medical Council in the UK that doctors can use off-label medication when there is sufficient evidence of the desired effect is met.

It is in the hope that more patients, and in particular those who have failed to gain relief with more "conventional" pain therapies, will get relief that a variety of drugs used in an "off-label" fashion will be presented.

PART 1

CHAPTER 4

Topical Nitrates

Every physician will be entirely familiar with the use of nitrates for their smooth muscle relaxant, and hence vasodilatory properties, in the treatment of ischemic heart disease. That when applied topically they can also have an analgesic and anti-inflammatory effect may be less well known.

It is well established that NSAIDs reduce inflammation and pain and hence they are extensively utilized in the management of soft tissue, joint, and postoperative pain. But with this promise of pain relief comes a very real risk of a variety of side effects that may preclude further use of an anti-inflammatory or even contraindicate its use in the first place. Since the incidence of pain from degenerative conditions and neoplasia increases with age as do the total or partial contraindications to the use of NSAIDs, a very real clinical problem may exist. It is for situations such as these that the possession of an effective alternative is needed and this can be at least partially filled by topically applied nitrates.

Mode of action of topical nitrates when used as analgesics

Nitric oxide (NO) is known to be a potent mediator in a variety of cellular systems such as the endothelium and both the peripheral and central nervous systems. It is released from the endothelium, neutrophils, and macrophages, all of which are known to be intimately involved in the inflammatory process. This release of NO from the endothelium is mimicked by exogenous nitrates such as glyceryl trinitrate (GTN) and isosorbide mononitrate (ISMN).

It appears that NO exerts its effect by stimulating increases in guanylate cyclase which causes an increase in the levels of 3'5'cyclic guanidine monophosphate (cGMP). Cholinergic drugs, such as acetylcholine, produce

Pain Management: Expanding the Pharmacological Options, Gary J. McCleane. © 2008 Blackwell Publishing, ISBN: 978-1-4051-7823-5.

analgesia in a similar fashion by releasing NO and increasing NO at nociceptor level. In addition to this action, NO may activate adenosine triphosphate (ATP) sensitive potassium channels and activate peripheral antinociception.

Human experimental pain

Little evidence is available from the literature of a pain-reducing effect of nitrates when administered to humans with induced pain. An isolated study does show that when nociceptive thresholds are measured using a pressure algometer the intravenous (IV) infusion of GTN increases the nociceptive threshold while infusion of placebo has no such effect.

Human clinical pain

In contrast to many of the therapeutic options available for pain treatment, the great weight of evidence of a potential analgesic effect comes from human clinical studies rather than from animal experimentation.

A variety of studies have shown a useful pain-reducing effect when topically applied GTN is compared to placebo. Among the conditions which have been investigated are:

- Infusion-related thrombophlebitis
- Supraspinatus tendonitis
- Ankle strain
- Achilles tendinopathy
- Extensor tendinosis (*Tennis Elbow*)
- Musculoskeletal pain
- Osteoarthritis
- Painful diabetic neuropathy
- Pain and inflammation after sclerosant injection for varicose veins.

What unifies many, but not all, of these conditions is the presence of localized pain, tenderness, and inflammation. The maximal effect of the topical nitrate is localized to the area of application. Effect is quick and may be apparent within an hour. Sustained use gives sustained relief and a number of studies have shown that after considerable periods of time the number of patients who have become asymptomatic is significantly higher in the nitrate-treated groups than in those treated with placebo. When topical GTN is used for the treatment of angina pectoris, it is advised that the patch is applied for 12 h on, 12 h off to prevent tachyphylaxis. The tolerance to the vasodilatory effect of this nitrate is not replicated when it is used for a pain relief and so the patch need only be changed once daily.

In those studies examining the effect of topical GTN on conditions where tissue inflammation is a significant and clearly visible process, application of GTN reduces the redness, swelling, and discomfort associated with the inflammatory process in a marked fashion.

Of course GTN is not the only nitrate. Isosorbide dinitrate (ISDN) is also extensively used in cardiological practice. In one study examining the pain associated with diabetic neuropathy, the spraying of ISDN onto the painful feet caused a reduction in the neuropathy pain. That said, diabetic neuropathy is a complex condition often associated with a degree of arterial and arteriolar disease that may cause tissue ischemia which could be lessened by the application of a vasodilatory substance such as GTN.

As well as an analgesic effect, nitrates clearly have a significant effect on smooth muscle. A significant and convincing literature now exists testifying to the beneficial effect of GTN ointment on anal fissures although whether this is merely due to the muscle relaxant effect of the nitrate as is conventionally stated or whether it could also be because of the analgesic effect of nitrate is open to speculation.

Effect of topical nitrates on analgesic effect of opioids

So far the use of a topical nitrate has been limited to its application for localized, often inflammatory pain. But it may also be that nitrates can have an effect on opioid analgesic tolerance. It has been suggested that endogenous NO may have some role in the analgesic tolerance seen with sustained opioid use and that therefore a synthetic NO donor such as GTN may have an effect on opioid-derived analgesia. In one study of patients taking morphine on a long-term basis for cancer-related pain, those patients co-treated with a GTN patch needed significantly less morphine to achieve adequate pain relief than those using a placebo patch. Similarly, when a GTN patch was used in patients who had received a spinal anesthetic containing the opioid sufentanil, the time to first request for additional analgesia was significantly longer than in those patients who used a placebo patch.

While few studies have been undertaken to examine the use of topical nitrates on opioid analgesia, it is at least reassuring that if one is using topical GTN for a localized pain and the patient is also taking an opioid then perhaps the nitrate will have the additional beneficial effect of augmenting the analgesic effect of the opioid.

Glyceryl trinitrate as a co-analgesic

Capsaicin, like GTN has a localized pain-relieving effect. The use of capsaicin is complicated by a burning discomfort and allodynia at the site of application which is often of a severity to preclude further use. When GTN is applied in combination with capsaicin three effects are apparent:

1 Individually both capsaicin and GTN have a local analgesic effect. When applied together, this effect is compounded.
2 The burning discomfort associated with capsaicin application is markedly reduced by co-application of GTN.
3 The allodynia caused by capsaicin application is significantly reduced by co-application of GTN.

Unresolved issues with the use of topical glyceryl trinitrate

1 Does the local analgesic effect demonstrated in the human studies in defined conditions have application to other currently unstudied conditions?
2 What is the optimal dose of GTN to achieve maximal pain relief and minimal side effects?
3 Does transdermal GTN augment all types of opioid-derived analgesia?
4 Do other nitrates have the same pain-relieving effects as GTN?

Glyceryl trinitrate formulations

GTN is produced in a range of formulations which include transdermal patches, ointments, sprays, tablets, and IV infusions. The vast majority of human pain studies have been with the patch formulations. These administer a measured and constant dose of the nitrate over a 24-h period. Currently patches are available which deliver approximately 5 or $10\,\text{mg}\,24\,\text{h}^{-1}$.

Perhaps one of the major problems with topical nitrate use is nitrate-associated headaches. These can be minimized if a small dose of nitrate is used. Often joint or soft tissue pain occurs in a number of sites and application at these differing sites would be desirable, but of course with more widespread use comes an increase of nitrate administered and hence an increased risk of headache. In practice, because smaller dose patches are not available, the commercially available patches can be cut into segments. This is only possible when the film-type patch (where the active drug is contained within the film) rather than the depot preparations (where a drug containing cream is enclosed in the patch by a semipermeable membrane) is used because if the latter is utilized, cutting the patch causes leakage of the drug containing cream. The ideal solution to these issues would be the availability of a GTN patch with a lower dosing rate.

The other formulation used in pain management is the ointment formulation. This is a greasy form which can stain adjacent clothes. Its major drawback is the inability to apply a measured and consistent dose.

Side effects of topical application of glyceryl trinitrate

As with all nitrates, headache is the most commonly encountered side effect associated with topical GTN use. This headache can be severe and the likelihood of its occurrence minimized by using as small a dose of GTN as is possible. Other side effects include a localized erythema at the patch application site and light-headedness. Because the potential analgesic effect of topical GTN is rapidly apparent, sustained use in the absence of relief is inappropriate.

Suggested clinical use

Mention has already been made of those conditions in which topical GTN has been shown in clinical trials to have a pain-relieving effect (See Figure 4.1). Anecdotal evidence would also suggest that topical GTN can reduce pain in, for example, the following conditions:

- Rheumatoid arthritis
- Ankylosing spondylitis
- Costochondritis
- Facet joint pain
- Fracture pain (particularly small bone fracture)
- Pathological fracture pain
- Ligament pain
- Enthetic pain
- Myofascial pain
- Postoperative wound pain
- Muscle pain
- Bursitis
- Coccidynia
- Complex regional pain syndrome type I pain
- Bony metastatic pain
- Pressure sore pain
- Vasculitic ulcer pain
- Vulvodynia
- Pain with peripheral vascular disease

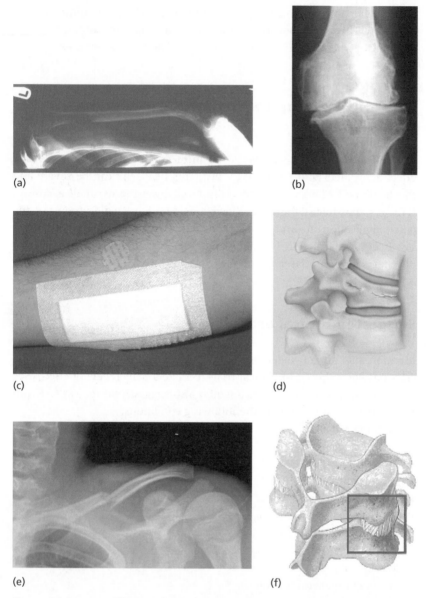

(a)   (b)

(c)   (d)

(e)   (f)

Figure 4.1 Some possible uses of topical GTN patches. (a) Metastatic deposit and pathological fracture. (b) Arthritic joint. (c) Postoperative wound. (d) Vertebral collapse fracture. (e) Bone fracture. (f) Facet joint pain.

When used for the like of fracture analgesia its particular merit arises where fracture stabilization (either internal or external) is impossible. For example, the application of a GTN patch over a fractured rib or over the site of a vertebral collapse fracture can be rewarded with useful pain relief and the patch may be used in isolation or along with other pharmacological options.

There are a number of situations in which topical GTN may be of particular benefit:

1 where pain is localized, has an inflammatory element, and is associated with local tissue tenderness;
2 where there is an incomplete analgesic response to NSAID or simple analgesic use;
3 where an NSAID is contraindicated (e.g., renal impairment, peptic ulcer disease, concurrent anticoagulant use);
4 where an increase in tissue perfusion may be beneficial;
5 with simple analgesics and NSAIDs before a stronger opioid is considered.

Conclusions

The topical application of GTN represents a simple, low-risk option for the treatment of localized pain. If this localized pain is associated with localized tenderness the chances of pain relief are increased. The risk of headache, the most common adverse effect associated with GTN use, can be minimized by using as small a dose of GTN as is possible. Because of the lack of effect of GTN on the renal, gastrointestinal and hematological systems, it can be used in place of NSAIDs when disorders of these systems exist when an NSAID may be contraindicated. Topical GTN can be used as a sole analgesic or in combination with other simple analgesics or NSAIDs.

Bibliography

Agrawal RP, Choudhary R, Sharma P et al. Glyceryl trinitrate spray in the management of painful diabetic neuropathy: a randomized double blind placebo controlled cross-over study. *Diabetes Res Clin Pract* 2007; 77: 494–5.

Berrazueta JR, Fleitas M, Salas E et al. Local transdermal glyceryl trinitrate has an anti-inflammatory action on thrombophlebitis induced by sclerosis of leg varicose veins. *Angiology* 1994; 45: 347–51.

Berrazueta JR, Losada A, Poveda J et al. Successful treatment of shoulder pain syndrome due to supraspinatus tendonitis with transdermal nitroglycerin. A double blind study. *Pain* 1996; 66: 63–7.

Devulder JE. Could nitric oxide be an important mediator in opioid tolerance and morphine side effects? *J Clin Anaesth* 2002; 14: 81–2.

Duarte ID, Lorenzetti BB, Ferreira SH. Acetylcholine induces peripheral analgesia by the release of nitric oxide. In: Moncada S and Higgs A (Eds), *Nitric oxide from L-arginine. A bioregulatory system.* Elsevier, Amsterdam, 1990; pp. 165–70.

Feelisch M, Noack EA. Correlation between nitric oxide formation during degradation of organic nitrates and activation of guanylate cyclase. *Eur J Pharmacol* 1987; 139: 19–30.

Knowles RG, Palacios M, Palmer RM, Moncada S. Formation of nitric oxide from L-arginine in the central nervous system: a transduction mechanism for stimulation of the soluble guanylate cyclase. *Proc Natl Acad Sci USA* 1989; 86: 5159–62.

Lauretti GR, de Oliveira R, Reis MP et al. Transdermal nitroglycerine enhances spinal sufentanil postoperative analgesia following orthopaedic surgery. *Anesthesiology* 1999; 90: 734–9.

Lauretti GR, Lima IC, Reis MP et al. Oral ketamine and transdermal nitroglycerin as analgesic adjuvant to oral morphine therapy for cancer pain management. *Anesthesiology* 1999; 90: 1528–33.

Lauretti GR, Perez MV, Reis MP, Pereira NL. Double-blind evaluation of transdermal nitroglycerine as an adjuvant to oral morphine for cancer pain management. *J Clin Anesth* 2002; 14: 83–6.

McCleane GJ. The addition of piroxicam to topically applied glyceryl trinitrate enhances its analgesic effect in musculoskeletal pain: a randomised, double-blind, placebo-controlled study. *Pain Clinic* 2000; 12: 113–6.

McCleane GJ. The analgesic efficacy of topical capsaicin is enhanced by glyceryl trinitrate in painful osteoarthritis: a randomized, double-blind, placebo controlled study. *Eur J Pain* 2000; 4: 355–60.

Okuda K, Sakurada C, Takahashi M et al. Characterization of nociceptive responses and spinal release of nitric oxide metabolites and glutamate evoked by different concentrations of formalin in rats. *Pain* 2001; 92: 107–15.

Paoloni JA, Appleyard RC, Nelson J, Murrell GA. Topical nitric oxide application in the treatment of chronic extensor tendinosis at the elbow: a randomized, double-blind, placebo-controlled clinical trial. *Am J Sports Med* 2003; 31: 915–20.

Paoloni JA, Appleyard RC, Nelson J, Murrell GA. Topical glyceryl trinitrate treatment of chronic noninsertional Achilles tendinopathy. A randomized, double-blind, placebo-controlled trial. *J Bone Joint Surg Am* 2004; 86: 916–22.

Paoloni JA, Appleyard RC, Nelson J, Murrell GA. Topical glyceryl trinitrate application in the treatment of chronic supraspinatus tendinopathy: a randomized, double-blinded, placebo-controlled clinical trial. *Am J Sports Med* 2005; 33: 806–13.

Soares A, Leite R, Tatsuo M, Duarte I. Activation of ATP sensitive K channels: mechanisms of peripheral antinociceptive action of the nitric oxide donor, sodium nitroprusside. *Eur J Pharmacol* 2000; 14: 67–71.

Thomsen LL, Brennum J, Iversen HK, Olesen J. Effect of a nitric oxide donor (glyceryl trinitrate) on nociceptive thresholds in man. *Cephalgia* 1996; 16: 169–74.

Yuen KC, Baker NR, Rayman G. Treatment of chronic painful diabetic neuropathy with isosorbide dinitrate spray: a double-blind placebo-controlled cross-over study. *Diabetes Care* 2002; 25: 1699–703.

CHAPTER 5

Topical Tricyclic Antidepressants

Few classes of drugs are more extensively used in the management of chronic pain conditions than the tricyclic antidepressants (TCAs). Substantial and convincing evidence supports their use in a variety of pain conditions including neuropathic pain and the pain associated with fibromyalgia. Their use is so common that it is now normal for them to be initiated by General Practitioners. The pain relief that may be apparent is independent of their antidepressant effects but any mood improvement that may occur is often welcome. In addition to pain reduction and mood improvement, muscle relaxation and normalization of sleep pattern may also occur. All oral TCA used for a pain indication is "off label."

Despite the widespread use of this class of drug in pain management, they are far from universally effective. Even when pain relief does occur, it is often partial. Indeed one would be more certain of an improvement in sleep with TCA use than pain reduction.

Among the side effects associated with oral TCA use are:
- Sleepiness
- Dry mouth
- Urinary retention
- Weight gain
- Paradoxical pain
- Palpitations

These side effects can be of a severity to reduce compliance and even when apparently well tolerated they may not contribute to a general feeling of well-being.

One is therefore left with a class of medication which a substantial and convincing body of evidence suggests are effective pain reducers for a variety of conditions but whose use in clinical practice is compromised by the frequent occurrence of side effects.

Pain Management: Expanding the Pharmacological Options, Gary J. McCleane. © 2008
Blackwell Publishing, ISBN: 978-1-4051-7823-5.

Mode of action of tricyclic antidepressants

It was initially supposed that TCAs reduced pain by augmenting the descending bulbospinal serotinergic and noradrenergic inhibitory drives. A pain signal arriving at the spinal cord is transmitted to the brain stem and thence to the cerebrum causing a downward signal that causes release of serotonin and noradrenaline/norepinephrine that inhibits further transmission of the pain signal from the spinal cord to the brain. It is now known that these actions do not fully explain the effects of TCAs and it is now thought that among the effects are those on the following structures and pathways:

- Descending bulbospinal serotinergic pathways
- Descending bulbospinal noradrenergic pathways
- NMDA receptors
- Opioid receptors
- Sodium channels
- Adenosine receptors

Of particular note are the last two, and probably the last three structures in this list. Sodium channels and adenosine receptors (and probably opioid receptors) have significant peripheral, as well as central, representation and so the possibility of a pain-reducing effect when applied by the topical route of administration exists for these drugs.

Experimental evidence

Adenosine receptors

At peripheral nerve terminals in rodents, adenosine A_1 receptor activation produces antinociception by decreasing, while adenosine A_2 receptor activation produces pronociception by increasing cyclic Adenosine Monophosphate (AMP) levels in the sensory nerve terminals. Adenosine A_3 receptor activation produces pain behaviors due to the release of histamine and 5HT from mast cells and subsequently activates the sensory nerve terminal. Caffeine acts as a non-specific adenosine receptor antagonist. When systemic caffeine is administered with systemic amitriptyline, the normal effect on thermal hyperalgesia is blocked. When amitriptyline is administered into a neuropathic paw, an antihyperalgesic effect is recorded (but not when it is given into the contralateral paw). This antihyperalgesic effect is blocked by caffeine, suggesting that at least part of the effect of peripherally applied amitriptyline is mediated through peripheral adenosine receptors.

Sodium channels

Sudoh and colleagues (2003) injected various TCAs by a single injection into rat sciatic notches. They measured the duration of complete sciatic nerve blockade and compared this with that of bupivicaine. They found that amitriptyline, doxepin, and imipramine produced a longer complete sciatic nerve block than bupivicaine whereas trimipramine and desipramine produced a shorter block. Nortriptyline and maprotiline failed to produce any block. When the effect of topical application of amitriptyline is compared with that of lidocaine, amitriptyline is seen to produce longer cutaneous analgesia than lidocaine.

These studies suggest, therefore, that from a mode of action perspective, TCAs could well have an analgesic effect when applied peripherally.

Animal evidence of an antinociceptive effect of peripherally applied TCAs

Neuropathic pain

A variety of experimentally induced neuropathic pain models exist. In one of these a constricting suture is applied around lumbar nerve roots which results in measurable signs of neuropathic pain such as allodynia and hyperalgesia. When amitriptyline is applied to rodent paws made neuropathic by a chronic nerve constriction injury, an antinociceptive effect is observed. When the amitriptyline is applied to the contralateral paw, no antinociceptive effect is observed in the paw on the injured side. When desipramine and the selective serotonin reuptake inhibitor (SSRI) fluoxetine are considered, desipramine has a similar antinociceptive effect when applied topically whereas fluoxetine does not.

Formalin test

The formalin test is a model of chronic inflammatory pain. Application of formalin to a rodent paw, for example, results in a biphasic response (the so-called first and second phase response) which can be measured electrophysiologically by recording the neural electrical response or by using behavioral tests such as observing the paw-licking response of the animal.

It seems that when amitriptyline and desipramine are co-administered peripherally with formalin, both the first and second phase responses are reduced.

When amitriptyline is administered peripherally along with formalin, Fos immunoreactivity in the dorsal region of the spinal cord is significantly lower than in animals where formalin is administered alone.

Thermal injury

Thermal hyperalgesia is produced by exposing a rodent hindpaw to 52°C for 45 s. Locally applied amitriptyline at the time of thermal injury produces both an antihyperalgesic and analgesic effects, depending on the concentration used. When the amitriptyline is applied after the injury the analgesic, but not antihyperalgesic, effect is retained.

Human pain

Paradoxically the human evidence for a pain-reducing effect with topical TCA application emerged before the animal work that verified the effect was published. Indeed, patients told clinicians that topical TCAs can reduce pain before clinicians hypothesized about this effect themselves. One remembers patients taking TCAs for a variety of uses telling us that when they had a toothache they held their TCA tablet against the offending tooth and that this reduced pain!

Human evidence of an analgesic effect with the topical application of TCAs is, however, limited but suggestive. A small randomized, placebo controlled trial (RCT) of 40 subjects with neuropathic pain of mixed etiology produced a reduction of 1.18 on a 0–10 linear visual analogue score (LVAS) relative to placebo use with the application of a doxepin 5% cream. Minor side effects were seen in only three subjects. A larger RCT involving 200 subjects, again with neuropathic pain of mixed etiology, suggested that 5% doxepin cream reduced LVAS by about one relative to placebo and that time to effect was about 2 weeks. Again side effects were minor and infrequent. A pilot study examining the effect of topical amitriptyline application failed to produce any pain relief, but the maximum therapy duration was 7 days and so the study may have been terminated before the time to maximal effect had been reached.

Case reports of a useful reduction in pain when 5% doxepin cream is applied topically in subjects with complex regional pain syndrome type I (CRPS) and when doxepin was used as an oral rinse in patients with oral pain as a result of cancer or cancer therapy have been made.

While the human evidence of an analgesic effect with topical doxepin is interesting, more study is needed to verify its, and other TCAs, effects when used by this route of administration. The evidence would suggest that the effect of topically applied doxepin is a local effect and that the consequences of systemic administration and hence systemic side effects can be substantially reduced.

It is suggested therefore that the topical application of a TCA represents a low-risk strategy for reducing pain and in contrast to the oral use of this type of medication, the risk of adverse effects associated with treatment are low.

Conditions which may benefit from topical TCA

The use of a topical TCA is only appropriate when the area over which pain is felt is relatively limited. If applied over too wide an area, systemic uptake will occur with an increased likelihood of systemic side effects. Uses are not limited just to neuropathic pain conditions:

* carpal tunnel syndrome	* meralgia paresthetica
* intercostal neuritis	* genitofemoral neuralgia
* ilioinguinal neuralgia	* supra and infraorbital neuritis
* postherpetic neuralgia	* painful diabetic neuropathy
* ulnar neuritis	* neuroma pain
* scar pain	* costochondritis
* enthetic pain	* muscle pain
* CRPS	* chemotherapy-related mucositis
* dysuria/urinary frequency	* coccidynia

The use of a topical TCA for urinary frequency and dysuria requires some explanation. In those who have to intermittently self-catheterize their bladders, dysuria and frequency can complicate repeated catheterization. If a TCA is applied to the tip of the urinary catheter, then these complications can be reduced.

Suggested clinical use

While no specific TCA containing preparation for topical application is specifically marketed for pain use, a commercially available variant is widely available for use in the treatment of the itch associated with eczema. This contains doxepin 5% in an aqueous base. When being used for pain relief a small amount is applied four times daily over the painful area with an expectation that between 2 and 3 weeks may pass before maximal pain relief is apparent. If over applied, then the side effects apparent with oral TCA use will become evident. Where a treatment plan is being considered for a patient, then this option would be at the simple end of the spectrum of complexities of therapy and would seem, where applicable, to be an easier option for the patient than either an oral TCA or antiepileptic drug.

While most human study has been with doxepin, some questions remain about the use of topical TCAs:

• Which TCA has the greatest analgesic effect when applied topically?
• What is the optimal dose and concentration of application to achieve maximal benefit?

It may be that use of a lower concentration of, for example, doxepin may allow a wider area of application without systemic side effects being produced and so allow its use in conditions where more widespread pain is experienced.

Bibliography

Epstein JB, Truelove EL, Oien H et al. Oral topical doxepin rinse: analgesic effect in patients with oral mucosal pain due to cancer or cancer therapy. *Oral Oncol* 2001; 37: 632–7.

Esser MJ, Chase T, Allen GV, Sawynok J. Chronic administration of amitriptyline and caffeine in a rat model of neuropathic pain: multiple interactions. *Eur J Pharmacol* 2001; 430: 211–18.

Esser MJ, Sawynok J. Acute amitriptyline in a rat model of neuropathic pain: differential symptom and route effects. *Pain* 1999; 80: 643–53.

Esser MJ, Sawynok J. Caffeine blockade of the thermal anti-hyperalgesic effect of acute amitriptyline in a rat model of neuropathic pain. *Eur J Pharmacol* 2000; 399: 131–9.

Haderer A, Gerner P, Kao G et al. Cutaneous analgesia after transdermal application of amitriptyline versus lidocaine in rats. *Anesth Analg* 2003; 96: 1707–10.

Heughan CE, Allen GV, Chase TD, Sawynok J. Peripheral amitriptyline suppresses formalin-induced Fos expression in the rat spinal cord. *Anesth Analg* 2002; 94: 427–31.

Lynch ME, Clarke AJ, Sawynok J. A pilot study examining topical amitriptyline, ketamine, and a combination of both in the treatment of neuropathic pain. *Clin J Pain* 2003; 19: 323–8.

McCleane GJ. Topical doxepin hydrochloride reduces neuropathic pain: a randomized, double-blind, placebo controlled study. *Pain Clinic* 1999; 12: 47–50.

McCleane GJ. Topical application of doxepin hydrochloride, capsaicin and a combination of both produces analgesia in chronic human neuropathic pain: a randomized, double-blind, placebo-controlled study. *Br J Clin Pharmacol* 2000; 49: 574–9.

McCleane GJ. Topical application of doxepin hydrochloride can reduce the symptoms of complex regional pain syndrome: a case report. *Injury* 2002; 33: 88–9.

McCleane GJ. Topical application of the tricyclic antidepressant doxepin can reduce dysuria and frequency. *Scandinavian J Urol Nephrol* 2004; 38: 88–9.

Oatway M, Reid A, Sawynok J. Peripheral antihyperalgesic and analgesic actions of ketamine and amitriptyline in a model of mild thermal injury in the rat. *Anesth Analg* 2003; 97: 168–73.

Pareek SS, Chopde CT, Thahus Desai PA. Adenosine enhances analgesic effect of tricyclic antidepressants. *Indian J Pharmacol* 1994; 26: 159–61.

Sawynok J. Adenosine receptor activation and nociception. *Eur J Pharmacol* 1998; 347: 1–11.

Sawynok J, Esser MJ, Reid AR. Peripheral antinociceptive actions of desipramine and fluoxetine in an inflammatory and neuropathic pain test in the rat. *Pain* 1999; 82: 149–58.

Sawynok J, Reid A. Peripheral interactions between dextromethorphan, ketamine and amitriptyline on formalin-evoked behaviours and paw edema in rats. *Pain* 2003; 102: 179–86.

Sawynok J, Reid AR, Esser MJ. Peripheral antinociceptive action of amitriptyline in the rat formalin test: involvement of adenosine. *Pain* 1999; 80: 45–55.

Sawynok J, Esser MJ, Reid AR. Antidepressants as analgesics: an overview of central and peripheral mechanisms of action. *J Psychiat Neurosci* 2001; 26: 21–9.

Su X, Gebhart GF. Effects of tricyclic antidepressants on mechanosensitive pelvic nerve afferent fibers innervating the rat colon. *Pain* 1998; 76: 105–14.

Sudoh Y, Cahoon EE, Gerner P, Wang GK. Tricyclic antidepressant as long acting local anesthetics. *Pain* 2003; 103: 49–55.

CHAPTER 6

Topical Opioids

The use of opioids of varying strengths is now a fundamental part of all aspects of pain management. The evidence supporting their use is impressive and increases with the passage of time. We now have opioids available in a wide range of formulations including several strong opioids in patch forms. When these are used the drug is administered transdermally with the aim of producing systemic concentrations of the drug to achieve central nervous system receptor activation. However, it is now becoming clear that the opioid receptors, at which opioids interact, are not only located in the central nervous system but also in peripheral nerve tissue. This being the case it may be that topically applied opioids may have a peripheral, as well as central, effect.

Peripheral opioid receptors

One method for examining the location of opioid receptors is to use autoradiographic techniques. When this technique is used in rats in which the sciatic nerve is ligated, opioid receptors are found to accumulate proximally and distally to the ligature in a time-dependent fashion suggesting that there is bidirectional axonal transport of these receptors. In another rodent model, non-inflamed paw tissue is known to contain some opioid receptors. When inflammation is induced by application of Freund's adjuvant to a paw, the density of opioid receptors increases in the paw massively. These opioid receptors are found in the cutaneous nerves and in immune cells infiltrating the surrounding tissue.

Using the same Freund's adjuvant model of inflammation, local injection of tumor necrosis factor or interleukin into the paw causes a dose-dependent increase in paw-pressure thresholds, or in other words a reduction in pain. This increase in paw-pressure thresholds is prevented

Pain Management: Expanding the Pharmacological Options, Gary J. McCleane. © 2008
Blackwell Publishing, ISBN: 978-1-4051-7823-5.

by local injection of the opioid antagonist naloxone and by the mu-opioid-specific antagonist CTOP (D-Phe-Cys-Tyr-D-Trp-Arg-Thr-Pen-Tr-NH$_2$). In animals pretreated with cyclosporin to suppress the immune system, the antinociceptive effect of the tumor necrosis factor is completely removed. It has been suggested, therefore, that cytokines release opioid peptides from immune cells of inflamed tissue, which act on opioid receptors present on sensory nerve terminals resulting in antinociception.

When DAMGO ([D-Ala(2),NMePhe(4), Gly(01)(S)],enkephalin), a mu-opioid ligand, is injected into tissue, the nociceptive effects of local irritant injection are reduced. In contrast, when DPDPE, a delta-opioid ligand is applied in a similar fashion, no change in nociception is observed. This suggests that peripheral mu-opioid receptors, and not delta-opioid receptors, are actively involved in nociceptive processing. Interestingly, in contrast to the central effect of opioids, there is a relative lack of antinociceptive tolerance to the effects of opioids on peripheral opioid receptors in inflamed tissue.

Topical opioids for pain

A number of clinical studies have been undertaken to examine the effect of peripherally applied opioids on pain. Methods of administration include the intra-articular injection of strong opioids used, for example, after knee arthroscopy. Two systematic reviews (1997 and 2001) have examined the evidence available at those times with one finding no effect, whereas the other found that intra-articular morphine given after knee arthroscopy had a definite analgesic effect. These reviews are now rather dated and may not reflect current evidence. In addition, even when a positive effect is apparent one is left with the question as to whether the effect is actually a local effect of the opioid or whether it represents the systemic uptake of the drug with a central effect. In addition, the animal evidence shows that opioid receptors migrate both proximally and distally to the nerve injury site or to the site of inflammation and this would clearly take time. In the human postoperative situation, enough time for peripheral migration of the opioid receptors to have occurred may not have passed and hence the equivocal results.

Some intriguing studies and case reports suggest that peripherally applied morphine can reduce pain. In one study, patients with painful mucositis following chemotherapy for head and neck carcinoma were studied. Patients received either a mouth rinse containing a local anesthetic or a rinse containing the local anesthetic and morphine. The duration of severe pain following chemotherapy was 3.5 days shorter and overall pain less severe in the morphine-treated group. It has also been shown in similar patients that a 2% morphine solution is more efficacious than a 1% solution. The average duration of relief after oral morphine rinse was 216 min. In these studies systemic morphine levels were measured, and even in the group who received morphine and obtained good relief, these levels were found to be insignificant.

In another study in patients with painful skin ulcers, those in whom the ulcer was washed out with 10 mg morphine obtained significantly more pain relief than those in whom the ulcers were washed out with saline.

Other studies have examined the effect of topical morphine on the pain following dental surgery. In one study, all patients had local anesthetic injected around the tooth socket after extraction. Half of them also had morphine applied to the socket. Patients were divided into those with/without inflammation. Injection of local anesthetic alone produced similar pain relief whether the surrounding tissue was inflamed or not. However, the morphine was more efficacious when applied to inflamed, rather than uninflamed, tissue. One is reminded of the increase in numbers of opioid receptors found in rat paws with induced inflammation compared to uninflamed paws.

A further potential use of peripherally applied opioids is in the management of bladder spasm which may complicate urological instrumentation. Case reports suggest that both morphine and diamorphine, when instilled intravesically, can produce relief without the occurrence of systemic side effects.

Conclusions

Animal models show that opioid receptors are found both peripherally and in the central nervous system. Indeed, following noxious insult, the density of peripheral opioid receptors increase and this may represent a target for peripherally applied opioids. The merit in such a use is that the troublesome side effects often found after systemic administration of opioids may be avoided. To date, the evidence of an effect in the clinical situation is relatively weak and hence further investigation is needed to confirm whether a definite effect is produced. From a practical perspective most practitioners are entirely happy with the use of opioids when administered systemically, and so if a situation arises where peripheral application seems to be worth considering, it could be argued that there is little to lose in trying this mode of application.

Bibliography

Cerchietti LC, Navigante AH, Bonomi MR et al. Effect of topical morphine for mucositis associated pain following concomitant chemo radiotherapy for head and neck carcinoma. *Cancer* 2002; 95: 2230–6.

Cerchietti LC, Navigante AH, Korte MW et al. Potential utility of the peripheral analgesic properties of morphine in stomatitis related pain. A pilot study. *Pain* 2003; 105: 265–73.

Coggeshall RE, Zhou S, Carlton SM. Opioid receptors on peripheral sensory axons. *Brain Res* 1997; 764: 126–32.

Czonkowski A, Stedin C, Herz A. Peripheral mechanisms of opioid antinociception in inflammation: involvement of cytokines. *Eur J Pharmacol* 1993; 242: 229–35.

Duckett JW, Cangiano T, Cubina M et al. Intravesical morphine analgesia after bladder surgery. *J Urol* 1997; 157: 1407–9.

Gupta A, Bodin L, Holmstrom B, Berggren L. A systematic review of the peripheral analgesic effects of intra articular morphine. *Anesth Analg* 2001; 93: 761–70.

Hassan AH, Ableitner A, Stein C, Herz A. Inflammation of the rat paw enhances axonal transport of opioid receptors in the sciatic nerve and increases their density in the inflamed tissue. *Neuroscience* 1993; 55: 185–95.

Krajnik M, Zylicz Z, Finlay I et al. Potential uses of topical opioids in palliative care – report of 6 cases. *Pain* 1999; 80: 121–5.

Likar R, Koppert W, Blatnig H et al. Efficacy of peripheral morphine analgesia in inflamed, non-inflamed and perineural tissue of dental surgery patients. *J Pain Symptom Manage* 2001; 21: 330–7.

Likar R, Sittl R, Gragger K et al. Peripheral morphine analgesia in dental surgery. *Pain* 1998; 76: 145–50.

McCoubrie R, Jeffrey D. Intravesical diamorphine for bladder spasm. *J Pain Symptom Manage* 2003; 25: 1–2.

Moore UJ, Seymour RA, Gilroy J, Rawlins MD. The efficacy of locally applied morphine in post-operative pain after bilateral third molar surgery. *Br J Clin Pharmacol* 1994; 37: 227–30.

Picard PR, Tramer MR, McQuay HJ, Moore RA. Analgesic efficacy of peripheral opioids (all except intra-articular): a qualitative systematic review of randomized controlled trials. *Pain* 1997; 72: 309–18.

Stein C, Machelska H, Binder W, Schafer M. Peripheral opioid analgesia. *Curr Opin Pharmacol* 2001; 1: 62–5.

Stein C, Machelska H, Schafer M. Peripheral analgesic and anti-inflammatory effects of opioids. *Z Rheumatol* 2001; 60: 416–24.

Stein C, Schafer M, Hassan AH. Peripheral opioid receptors. *Ann Med* 1995; 27: 19–21.

Twillman RK, Long TD, Cathers TA, Mueller DW. Treatment of painful skin ulcers with topical opioids. *J Pain Symptom Manage* 1999; 17: 288–92.

Zeppetella G, Paul J, Ribeiro MD. Analgesic efficacy of morphine applied topically to painful ulcers. *J Pain Symptom Manage* 2003; 25: 555–8.

Zhou L, Zhang Q, Stein C, Schafer M. Contribution of opioid receptors on primary afferent versus sympathetic neurons to peripheral opioid analgesia. *J Pharmacol Exp Ther* 1998; 286: 1000–6.

CHAPTER 7
Topical Local Anesthetics

The concept of applying a locally active agent to the site of pain in the hope of achieving pain relief is both appealing and in many cases achievable. And yet to date only lidocaine 5% patches have a formal indication for use in pain treatment with that being for use in postherpetic neuralgia. Therefore, in practice, the use of topical local anesthetics for local pain relief is common with that use being largely "off-label".

The mechanism of the analgesic action of local anesthetic agents appears to be related to the ability of these agents to reduce the activity of peripheral sodium channels within sensory afferents with subsequent reduction of ectopic, paroxysmal discharges and ultimate reduction of pain transmission. The use of local anesthetic agents as analgesic agents in fact has been associated with reduced expression of mRNA for certain types of sodium channels. A separate mechanism of action of the lidocaine 5% patch may be that the patch itself may serve to protect allodynia skin. Different local anesthetic preparations may have different effects with respect to the manner in which they create analgesia. For example, the lidocaine 5% patch produces its analgesic effect without causing anesthesia; in contrast, the use of EMLA cream (eutectic mixture of local anesthetics, 2.5% lidocaine/2.5% prilocaine) may result in a clearly demonstrable anesthetic effect on the skin to which it is applied. Consequently, these differences may lead one to use EMLA cream for acute painful states such as venipuncture, lumbar puncture, intramuscular injections, and operative pain in the like of circumcision.

Lidocaine 5% patch

For almost a decade a patch containing 5% lidocaine has been available in the US of America for topical use in patients with postherpetic

---

Pain Management: Expanding the Pharmacological Options, Gary J. McCleane. © 2008
Blackwell Publishing, ISBN: 978-1-4051-7823-5.

neuralgia. This patch has recently received a marketing authorization in the UK with a similar indication for postherpetic neuralgia. Significant experience with use of topical lidocaine 5% patches suggests that they effectively produce analgesia in a variety of pain con-ditions as well as in the accepted use in postherpetic neuralgia. For example, rand-omized controlled trials have shown that this patch can reduce periph-eral neuropathic pain (where the "numbers needed to treat," NNT is 4.4) and neuropathic pain of mixed etiology. Case report and open-label studies have also suggested that it can be utilized in the treatment of carpal tunnel syndrome, idiopathic sensory polyneuropathy, low back pain, painful diabetic neuropathy, osteoarthritis, and myofascial pain (Table 7.1).

From a practical perspective, a topical lidocaine patch is worth consider-ation whenever there is an area of allodynia which the patch can cover or there is a relatively localized area of tenderness. The etiology of the allody-nia or tenderness is unimportant. Time to effect is measured in hours and so a prolonged trial period is not necessary. If required several patches can be used concurrently.

One example of the use of lidocaine 5% patch is in the treatment of rib fracture. This acutely painful condition is not only unpleasant for the patient but may also impair respiratory function to the extent that pul-monary complications may result. Conventional treatment includes the use of simple, compound, and strong analgesics, NSAIDs, and where these are insufficient, the use of intercostal nerve blocks and thoracic epi-dural injections. Clinical experience indicates that application of lidocaine 5% patch to the fracture site either alone, or in combination with oral

Table 7.1 Potential uses of lidocaine 5% patch.

Postherpetic neuralgia	
Peripheral neuropathic pain*	Postoperative pain**
Neuropathic pain of mixed etiology*	Carpal tunnel syndrome**
	Idiopathic sensory polyneuropathy**
	Painful diabetic neuropathy**
	Low back pain**
	Myofascial syndrome**
	Osteoarthritis**
	Fracture pain (e.g., rib fracture)**
	Tendonitis**
	CRPS**
	Neuroma pain**
	Ligament pain**

*Use suggested by randomized controlled trial.
**Use suggested by case report/open-label studies/clinical experience.

analgesics is often rewarded with significant pain reductions so that more aggressive forms of treatment are unnecessary.

The manufacturers recommend that the patch be used 12 h on, 12 h off, presumably to minimize the risk of systemic absorption. It is suggested that this is not necessary and that 24-h use with daily application is entirely appropriate. As we will see later in the chapter on intravenous (IV) lidocaine, the worry about systemic absorption is greatly overplayed.

Perhaps one of the greatest fears with the use of topical lidocaine may be that the sustained use of this drug, even when applied topically, may allow systemic concentrations to increase above the level at which systemic side effects may occur. In reality, Lidocaine 5% patch contains approximately 700 mg of lidocaine of which around only 5% is released. When applied topically for 12 h on, 12 h off in the treatment of postherpetic neuralgia, the highest concentration found after single patch use in one study was $0.1 \mu gl^{-1}$, whereas when four patches were applied for 18 h daily to volunteers, the peak systemic lidocaine levels reached were $0.153 \mu gl^{-1}$. These levels are significantly below those which would be associated with systemic side effects. In another study the levels of both lidocaine and monoethylglycinexylidide, the primary active metabolite of lidocaine were found to be negligible. It seems, therefore, that systemic toxicity is not a potential complication of lidocaine 5% use.

Gels/creams

Several topical local anesthetic preparations are available in gel and cream form. Amethocaine is available as a gel and lidocaine/prilocaine are presented as "EMLA®" cream. EMLA® cream contains a eutectic mixture of lidocaine and prilocaine and its use has become established in the anesthetizing of skin prior to cannula insertion. It also has demonstrable benefit in reducing the pain of other procedures including lumbar puncture, intramuscular injections, and circumcision. While EMLA® cream is not USFDA approved for any neuropathic pain condition, several studies have been undertaken in patients with postherpetic neuralgia. Two of these were uncontrolled and showed a pain-reducing effect, while a randomized controlled study in the same condition failed to show any benefit. Caution should be used with long-term use of this preparation as prilocaine use has been associated with the onset of methaemoglobinaemia.

Other topical local anesthetics

While lidocaine patch, EMLA cream, and amethocaine gel have received most attention, they are not the only way of using a peripherally applied local anesthetic to reduce pain. One variant on topical lidocaine use is the use of a liposomal lidocaine preparation which enhances dermal penetration to allow a quicker onset of action (Maxilene®, RGR Pharma, Windsor, Ont). This would be of benefit for the management of incident pain such as venipuncture.

While we conventionally use the term "local anesthetic" to indicate drugs like lidocaine, prilocaine, and bupivicaine, for example, it also implies a sodium channel blocking effect as the mode of action. A wide variety of other drugs also have a sodium channel blocking effect (e.g., some of the antiepileptic drugs, membrane stabilizers such as mexiletine). One of the classes of drugs that have among their mode of action a sodium channel blocking effect are the tricyclic antidepressants. As we have seen in Chapter 5, the tricyclic antidepressant doxepin has been shown to have a pain-reducing effect when applied topically and at least some of this effect may be apportioned to its effects on sodium channels. One of the case reports that suggest that doxepin can have a topical effect describes its use in patients following chemoradiotherapy for head and neck cancer who developed painful mucositis. Mouth washes with doxepin caused useful pain reduction. Another drug useful in this situation is cocaine. Originally used in medical practice by the father of psychoanalysis, Sigmund Freud, who was also an ophthalmologic surgeon, who applied it topically to the cornea to produce corneal anesthesia, can also have a role in the management of painful mucositis. From a practical perspective, it can be frozen in the form of a lolly pop, with or without flavoring such as orange, to achieve oral anesthesia to reduce the pain from the mucositis.

Conclusion

There is a logical appeal to applying a locally active agent to the site where pain is felt. While lidocaine 5% patch has postherpetic neuralgia as its indication, common sense would suggest that it has potential value in any pain condition where the pain is relatively localized, regardless of whether the pain is neuropathic or not. Because systemic absorption of the lidocaine from the patch, even with sustained use, is minimal, the risks associated with lidocaine patch use are minimal. While there is also logic to the use of local anesthetic creams and gels, their merit is in acute use to anesthetize skin and other tissue rather than in longer-term use as a method of pain control.

One could speculate that alternative concentrations of lidocaine in a patch formulation may optimize the pain relief apparent in various clinical scenarios and further investigation is warranted.

Bibliography

Argoff CE. Conclusions: chronic pain studies of lidocaine patch 5% using the neuropathic pain scale. *Curr Med Res Opin* 2004; 20 (Suppl 2): S29–31.

Argoff CE, Galer BS, Jensen MP et al. Effectiveness of the lidocaine patch 5% on pain qualities in three chronic pain states: assessment with the neuropathic pain scale. *Curr Med Res Opin* 2004; 20 (Suppl): S21–8.

Attal N, Brasseur L, Chauvin M. Effects of single and repeated applications of a eutectic mixture of local anesthetics (EMLA®) cream on spontaneous and evoked pain in post-herpetic neuralgia. *Pain* 1999; 81: 203–9.

Barbano RL, Herrmann DN, Hart-Gouleau S et al. Effectiveness, tolerability, and impact on quality of life of the 5% lidocaine patch in diabetic polyneuropathy. *Arch Neurol* 2004; 61: 914–18.

Campbell BJ, Rowbotham M, Davis PS et al. Systemic absorption of topical lidocaine in normal volunteers, patients with post-herpetic neuralgia, and patients with acute herpes zoster. *J Pharm Sci* 2002; 91: 1343–50.

Dalpiaz AS, Dodds TA. Myofascial pain response to topical lidocaine therapy: case report. *J Pain Palliat Care Pharmacother* 2002; 16: 99–104.

Dalpiaz AS, Lordon SP, Lipman AG. Topical lidocaine patch therapy for myofascial pain. *J Pain Palliat Care Pharmacother* 2004; 18: 15–34.

Galer BS, Gammaitoni AR, Oleka N et al. Use of the lidocaine patch 5% in reducing intensity of various pain qualities reported by patients with low-back pain. *Curr Med Res Opin* 2004; 20 (Suppl): S5–12.

Galer BS, Jensen MP, Ma T et al. The lidocaine patch 5% effectively treats all neuropathic pain qualities: results of a randomized, double-blind, vehicle-controlled, 3-week efficacy study with use of the neuropathic pain scale. *Clin J Pain* 2002; 18: 297–301.

Galer BS, Rowbotham MC, Perander J, Friedman E. Topical lidocaine patch relieves postherpetic neuralgia more effectively than a vehicle topical patch: results of an enriched enrolment study. *Pain* 1999; 80: 533–8.

Gammaitoni AR, Davis MW. Pharmacokinetics and tolerability of lidocaine patch 5% with extended dosing. *Ann Pharmacother* 2002; 36: 236–40.

Gammaitoni AR, Galer BS, Onawola R et al. Lidocaine patch 5% and its positive impact on pain qualities in osteoarthritis: results of a pilot 2-week, open-label study using the neuropathic pain scale. *Curr Med Res Opin* 2004; 20 (Suppl): S13–19.

Gimbel J, Linn R, Hale M, Nicholson B. Lidocaine patch treatment in patients with low back pain: results of an open-label, nonrandomized pilot study. *Am J Ther* 2005; 12: 311–19.

Herrmann DN, Barbano RL, Hart-Gouleau S et al. An open-label study of the lidocaine patch 5% in painful idiopathic sensory polyneuropathy. *Pain Med* 2005; 6: 379–84.

Hines R, Keaney D, Moskowitz MH, Prakken S. Use of lidocaine patch 5% for chronic low back pain: a report of four cases. *Pain Med* 2002; 3: 361–5.

Litman SJ, Vitkun SA, Poppers PJ. Use of EMLA® cream in the treatment of post-herpetic neuralgia. *J Clin Anesth* 1996; 8: 54–7.

Lycka BA, Watson CP, Nevin K et al. EMLA® cream for the treatment of pain caused by post-herpetic neuralgia: a double-blind, placebo controlled study. In: Proceedings of the annual meeting of the American Pain Society 1996: A111 (abstract).

McCleane GJ. Topical analgesics. *Med Clin N Am* 2007; 91: 125–39.

Meier T, Wasner G, Faust M et al. Efficacy of lidocaine patch 5% in the treatment of focal peripheral neuropathic pain syndromes: a randomized, double-blind, placebo-controlled study. *Pain* 2003; 106: 151–8.

Nalamachu S, Crockett RS, Gammaitoni AR, Gould EM. A comparison of the lidocaine patch 5% vs naproxen 500 mg twice daily for the relief of pain associated with carpal tunnel syndrome: a 6-week randomized, parallel-group study. *MedGenMed* 2006; 8: 33.

Nalamachu S, Crockett RS, Mathur D. Lidocaine patch 5% for carpal tunnel syndrome: how it compares with injections: a pilot study. *J Fam Pract* 2006; 55: 209–14.

Rowbotham MC, Davies PS, Verkempinck C, Galer BS. Lidocaine patch: double-blind controlled study of a new treatment for post-herpetic neuralgia. *Pain* 1996; 65: 39–44.

Taddio A, Soin HK, Schuh S, Koren G et al. Liposomal lidocaine to improve procedural success rates and reduce procedural pain among children: a randomized controlled trial. *CMAJ* 2005; 172: 1691–5.

CHAPTER 8

Topical Glutamate Receptor Antagonists

Within the dorsal spinal cord, both ionotropic glutamate receptors (N-methyl-D-aspartate, NMDA), α-amino-3-hydroxy-5-methyl-4-isoxazolepropionic acid (AMPA), kainic acid (KA) and metabotropic glutamate receptors are involved in nociceptive signaling and central sensitization in chronic pain conditions. Both the systemic and spinal administration of multiple classes of glutamate receptor antagonists have been observed to produce analgesia in a variety of persistent pain models, and although their potential as analgesics has been investigated, they have a tendency to produce unacceptable side effects. Perhaps the most extensively used glutamate receptor antagonist in human practice is ketamine.

More recently it has been appreciated that multiple glutamate receptors are also expressed on peripheral nerve terminals, and that these may contribute to peripheral nociceptive signaling (Table 8.1).

Table 8.1 Excitatory and inhibitory influences on peripheral nerve activity by mediators released by tissue injury and inflammation and by agents acting on neuroreceptors.

Inhibitory influences	Excitatory influences
Opioids (μ, δ, κ)	Prostanoids (EP, IP)
GABA (GABA$_B$)	α_2-adrenoreceptor (α_{2A})
α_2-adrenoreceptor (α_{2C})	Bradykinin (B$_1$, B$_2$)
Orphinan (ORL$_1$)	Glutamate (NMDA, AMPA, KA)
Adenosine (A$_1$)	Histamine (H$_1$)
Somatostatin	Acetylcholine (N)
Cannabinoids (CB$_1$, CB$_2$)	Serotonin (5HT$_1$, 5HT$_2$, 5HT$_3$, 5HT$_4$)
	Adenosine (A$_{2A}$, A$_3$)
	ATP (P2X$_3$)
	Tachykinins (NK$_1$, NK$_2$)
	Nerve growth factor (TrkA)

Pain Management: Expanding the Pharmacological Options, Gary J. McCleane. © 2008 Blackwell Publishing, ISBN: 978-1-4051-7823-5.

Ionotropic and metabotropic glutamate receptors are present on membranes of unmyelinated peripheral axons and axon terminals in the skin, and peripheral inflammation increases the proportions of both unmyelinated and myelinated nerves expressing ionotropic glutamate receptors. Local injections of NMDA and non-NMDA glutamate receptor agonists to the rat hindpaw or knee joint enhance pain behaviors generating hyperalgesia and allodynia. Intraplanter injection of metabotropic glutamate receptor agonists produces similar actions. On the contrary, local administration of antagonists of both ionotropic and metabotropic receptors inhibits pain behavior evoked by kaolin and carrageenan injected into the knee joint.

Inflammation of the hindpaw or the knee joint produces a local release of glutamate that appears to originate from A and C fibers. An additional indirect mechanism, via activation of glutamate receptors on sympathetic afferents to release norepinephrine and other substances from postganglionic efferents (e.g., ATP, neuropeptide Y), can occur as NMDA, AMPA, and KA receptors are also present on postganglionic sympathetic efferents, and inflammation enhances the expression of such receptors. Collectively, these results suggest that the involvement of local release of glutamate receptors and activation of both ionotropic and metabotropic glutamate receptors in inflammatory pain in particular, and raises the possibility that peripheral application or possibly topical formulations of such agents may be useful as analgesics. Whether topical application results in sufficient dermal transfer of the drug or whether intradermal or subcutaneous injection is required is not yet clear. It is also possible that peripheral glutamate receptors play a significant role in peripheral pain signaling in neuropathic pain (as occurs at spinal sites), but this contention is as yet unsubstantiated.

Human evidence

In a thermal injury model in healthy human volunteers, subcutaneous injection of ketamine is reported to produce a long-lasting reduction in hyperalgesia in one study, while in another produced only short-term pain relief with no effect on hyperalgesia. When capsaicin is injected intradermally as an irritant, peripherally administered ketamine has no effect on the pain produced. It may be, therefore, that peripherally applied ketamine's effect is dependent on which type of tissue irritation has occurred. Then again, ketamine is not only active on glutamate receptors, having also local anesthetic effects, blocks calcium channels, alters cholinergic and monoaminergic actions, and interacts with opioid mechanisms, and any effect apparent after peripheral application may be due to any one or all of these other effects. The peripheral contribution of glutamate receptors to pain may be more pronounced in conditions involving chronic inflammation where up-regulation of receptors occurs, or in conditions involving nerve injury. In humans, it is reported that the synovial fluid of arthritic patients has an elevated glutamate and aspartate content.

Several human clinical studies have suggested that peripherally applied ketamine can have analgesic effects. For example, when the peritonsillar area is infiltrated with ketamine prior to tonsillectomy, lower pain scores are recorded than when placebo is used. When compared to administration of a similar dose of ketamine intravenously, similar pain reductions are seen, but significantly less sedation is encountered when the drug is injected into the peritonsillar region than when given intravenously. Similarly, when ketamine is injected subcutaneously prior to circumcision, significantly less pain is experienced than when saline is injected. Of course, this may be a result of systemic uptake of the agent or represent an effect generated by one of the other modes of action of ketamine rather than its glutamate receptor effect.

It seems, therefore, that there is animal evidence to suggest that peripherally applied glutamate receptor antagonists may have a pain-reducing effect but as yet the clinical significance of these findings has not been established. As well as the conundrum about whether glutamate receptor antagonists have an analgesic effect by virtue of their peripheral effect, there are also issues concerning how well peripherally applied, and in particular topically applied, antagonist may be absorbed so as to have an effect on the receptors. Perhaps localized injection is needed. Even if peripheral application is successful in reducing pain the human experimental evidence would suggest that this effect is dependent on the type of pain in question.

Bibliography

Bhave G, Karim F, Carlton SM, Fereau RW. Peripheral group I metabotropic glutamate receptors modulate nociception in mice. *Nat Neurosci* 2001; 4: 417–23.

Carlton SM. Peripheral excitatory amino acids. *Curr Opin Pharmacol* 2001; 1: 52–6.

Carlton SM, Coggeshall RE. Inflammation-induced changes in peripheral glutamate receptor populations. *Brain Res* 1999; 820: 63–70.

Carlton SM, Hargett GL, Coggeshall RE. Localization and activation of glutamate receptors in unmyelinated axons of rat glabrous skin. *Neurosci Lett* 1995; 197: 25–8.

Coderre TJ, Katz J, Vaccarino A, Melzack R. Contribution of central neuroplasticity to pathological pain: review of clinical and experimental evidence. *Pain* 1993; 52: 259–85.

Dal C, Celebi N, Elvan EG et al. The efficacy of intravenous (IV) or peritonsillar infiltration of ketamine for postoperative pain relief in children following adenotonsillectomy. *Paediatr Anaesth* 2007; 17: 263–9.

Davidson EM, Carlton SM. Intraplantar injection of dextromethorphan, ketamine or memantine attenuates formalin-induced behaviours. *Brain Res* 1998; 785: 136–42.

Davidson EM, Coggeshall RE, Carlton SM. Peripheral NMDA and non-NMDA glutamate receptors contribute to nociceptive behaviours in the rat formalin test. *Neuroreport* 1997; 8: 941–6.

De Groot K, Zhou S, Carlton SM. Peripheral glutamate release in the hindpaw following low and high intensity sciatic stimulation. *Neuroreport* 2000; 11: 497–502.

Fisher K, Coderre TJ, Hagen NA. Targeting the N-methyl-D-aspartate receptor for chronic pain management: preclinical animal studies, recent clinical experience and future research direction. *J Pain Symptom Manage* 2000; 20: 358–73.

Hirota K, Lambert DG. Ketamine: its mechanisms of action and unusual clinical uses. *Br J Anaesth* 1996; 77: 441–4.

Jackson DL, Graff CB, Richardson JD, Hargreaves KM. Glutamate participates in the peripheral modulation of thermal hyperalgesia in rats. *Eur J Pharmacol* 1995; 284: 321–5.

Lawland NB, McNearney T, Westlund KN. Amino acid release into the knee joint: key role in nociception and inflammation. *Pain* 2000; 86: 69–74.

McNearney T, Speegle D, Lawland N et al. Excitatory amino acid profiles of synovial fluid from patients with arthritis. *J Rheumatol* 2000; 27: 739–45.

Omote K, Kawamata T, Kawamata M, Namiki A. Formalin-induced release of excitatory amino acids in the skin of the rat hindpaw. *Brain Res* 1998; 787: 161–4.

Pedersen JL, Galle TS, Kehlet H. Peripheral analgesic effects of ketamine in acute inflammatory pain. *Anesthesiology* 1998; 89: 58–66.

Sawynok J, Reid AR. Modulation of formalin-induced behaviours and edema by local and systemic administration of dextromethorphan, memantine and ketamine. *Eur J Pharmacol* 2002; 450: 153–62.

Tan PH, Cheng JT, Kuo CH et al. Preincisional subcutaneous infiltration of ketamine suppresses postoperative pain after circumcision surgery. *Clin J Pain* 2007; 23: 214–18.

Tverskoy M, Oren M, Vaskovich M et al. Ketamine enhances local anesthetic and analgesic effects of bupivicaine by a peripheral mechanism: a study in postoperative patients. *Neurosci Lett* 1996; 215: 5–8.

Walker K, Reeve A, Bowes M, et al. mGlu5 receptors and nociceptive function II. mGlu5 receptors functionally expressed on peripheral sensory neurons mediate inflammatory hyperalgesia. *Neuropharmacology* 2001; 40: 10–19.

Warncke T, Jorum E, Stubhaug A. Local treatment with the N-methyl-D-aspartate receptor antagonist ketamine, inhibits development of secondary hyperalgesia in man by a peripheral action. *Neurosci Lett* 1997; 227: 1–4.

Zhou S, Bonasera L, Carlton SM. Peripheral administration of NMDA, AMPA or KA results in pain behaviours in rats. *Neuroreport* 1996; 7: 895–900.

Zhou S, Komak S, Du J, Carlton SM. Metabotropic glutamate 1α receptors on peripheral primary afferent fibers: their role in nociception. *Brain Res* 2001; 913: 18–26.

CHAPTER 9

Topical, Oral, and Perineural α-Adrenoreceptor Agonists

Perhaps the most extensive use of α-adrenoreceptor antagonists is in anesthesiological practice. However, examination of the emerging literature, both of a clinical and preclinical nature, suggests that use of agents active on these receptors may have much wider clinical applications.

Normally sympathetic mechanisms do not cause excitation of primary afferent neurons. However, following experimentally induced nerve injury the following effects are noted:

- coupling occurs between sympathetic fibers and afferent terminals in the neuroma following nerve cut or ligation, and sympathetic stimulation or norepinephrine can cause excitation of unmyelinated nerves,
- coupling occurs between unlesioned postganglionic and afferent nerve terminals following partial nerve lesions, and
- sympathetic nerve terminals enter the dorsal root ganglia and form basket-like structures around dorsal root ganglia cell bodies, particularly larger diameter cells, providing a collateral innervation from sympathetic terminals that normally supply blood vessels.

Thus sympathetic-afferent coupling occurs at three distinct sites; at the site of injury, at the sensory terminal, and within dorsal root ganglia. The relative contributions of these mechanisms to sympathetic-afferent coupling in the different nerve injury conditions are highly dependent on the location and nature of the lesion as well as the time following injury.

Both behavioral and electrophysiological studies indicate that α_2-adrenoreceptors are primary mediators of sympathetic-afferent coupling following nerve injury. Multiple α_2-adrenoreceptors have been detected in rat dorsal root ganglia, with α_{2C} on most, α_{2A} on some, and α_{2B} on few neurons. Nerve ligation or transection results in an up-regulation of α_{2A}-adrenoreceptors, and a decrease or no change in α_{2C}-adrenoreceptors in rat dorsal root ganglia. Afferent excitation following nerve injury

Pain Management: Expanding the Pharmacological Options, Gary J. McCleane. © 2008
Blackwell Publishing, ISBN: 978-1-4051-7823-5.

is thought to result from α_{2A}-adrenoreceptor activation. The α_1-adrenoreceptors are also involved in such activation in some conditions.

The sympathetic nervous system also contributes to hyperalgesia following tissue injury and inflammation, but the nature of the involvement in this case differs from that in nerve injury. Inflammation does not lead to up-regulation of α_{2A}-adreneoreceptors in dorsal root ganglia, and in this case, the enhancing effect of norepinephrine on the sensitivity of primary afferents may be mediated indirectly by actions on sympathetic postganglionic nerves. The α_2-adrenoreceptor activation can also produce analgesia following localized administration in an inflammatory model. Hyperalgesia is proposed to be mediated by α_{2B}-adrenoreceptors located on sympathetic postganglionic neurons, and analgesia by α_{2C}-adrenoreceptors on primary afferent terminals. The α_{2C}-receptor on primary afferents may exist as part of a tri-receptor complex along with mu-opioid and adenosine A_1 receptors.

The presence and importance of α-adrenoreceptors at or near the site of nerve injury or inflammation is further confirmed by the reduction in pain and hypersensitivity seen when α-adrenoreceptor agonists such as clonidine are administered and the abolition of this effect seen when α-adrenoreceptors antagonists such as BRL44408 are given. Not only does clonidine reduce hypersensitivity and pain but it also reduces the secretion of cytokines such as interleukin 6 and interleukin 1 beta at the site of injury.

Clinical use of α-adrenoreceptor agonists

In human practice two α-adrenoreceptor agonists are widely available. These are clonidine and tizanadine. Clonidine is produced in a patch, oral, and injectable formulations, whereas tizanadine is available as an oral preparation.

Although tizanadine is marketed as a drug that reduces muscle spasm, but which may also have analgesic properties, many more uses are attributed to clonidine:
- Can augment the quality and duration of effect of local anesthetics
- Can act as a sole analgesic
- Can reduce the symptoms of an opioid withdrawal reaction

Prolongation of local anesthetic effect
Local anesthetics are widely used particularly in perioperative pain management when they are infiltrated around operative wounds, are used in nerve blocks, and are used by the epidural and intrathecal routes.

An intriguing study in human volunteers has shown that co-administration of clonidine with lidocaine prolongs the anesthetic effect of the lidocaine. In this study, 0.5% lidocaine was injected subcutaneously into one forearm, while an equal volume of lidocaine 0.5% along with 10 μg of clonidine was injected subcutaneously into the other. The mean time to return of normal sensation as measured using pin pricks was 3.5 h in the lidocaine only injected skin as opposed to 6 h in the lidocaine and clonidine injected side. While infiltration of the area around a postoperative wound often gives good pain relief, this is of finite duration with the cessation of effect often occurring after hospital discharge. If the same effect is apparent when clonidine is added to longer acting local anesthetics such as bupivicaine, then there would be a very real chance that quality of postoperative pain management of these patients could be significantly enhanced. Given that addition of clonidine to bupivicaine and ropivicaine does enhance the effects of these local anesthetics when used for nerve blocks, then it seems highly likely that this effect would be replicated when used for skin infiltration.

This apparent peripheral effect of clonidine is mirrored by a further study where bupivicaine alone was instilled into the abdominal cavity alone or in combination with clonidine in patients undergoing total abdominal hysterectomy with those having the clonidine being found to have a significantly longer period before their first request for supplemental pain relief.

Clonidine can also be co-administered with a local anesthetic when undertaking a nerve block or epidural for the purposes of postoperative pain relief. When clonidine is used in this fashion it can be given either, along with the local anesthetic, as a single shot with the expectation that it will prolong the pain relieving effect of the block or as a continuous infusion. When given as a continuous infusion, the hope is that the quality of pain relief produced is enhanced or that a similar level of analgesia is apparent, despite the fact that a lower concentration of local anesthetic is used. If, for example, in the case of epidural pain relief for laboring mothers, the use of a lower concentration of local anesthetic increases the chances of the mother remaining ambulant, particularly during the earlier stages of the labor. Perhaps the major drawback of continual infusion of clonidine is the hypotension and sedation that may complicate its use.

When clonidine is given along with a local anesthetic for a peripheral nerve block, its effect may be peripheral as well as central. In one study of volunteers who received a brachial block with local anesthetic with or without clonidine or an intramuscular injection of a similar dose of clonidine or saline, the addition of clonidine to the brachial blocking injectate significantly prolonged the duration of block and produced much lower systemic concentrations of clonidine than did the intramuscular injection. When clonidine was given intramuscularly, there was no prolongation of the duration of brachial block produced by a local anesthetic alone.

Clonidine as a sole analgesic

A number of studies show that both oral and transdermally applied clonidine can reduce the pain of migraine, facial pain, and Complex Regional Pain Syndrome (CRPS), for example. The major impediment to the use of clonidine by the oral or transdermal route is the side effects associated with systemic clonidine use. Hypotension, sedation, and dry mouth are common with clonidine use. Indeed, in the past, a major use of clonidine was in the management of hypertension. Where clonidine comes into its own is when it is given by the epidural route when a single injection of, for example, 150 μg can produce pain relief whose duration is measured in weeks and, on occasions, months. This clonidine can be given by a conventional lumbar epidural injection or by the caudal epidural route. While light-headedness and sedation are frequent complications of epidural use, these side effects last up to 12 h in contrast to the pain relief that can last many weeks. The analgesic effect produced can be for pain in any region of the body and not just the segmental level at which the epidural injection is given. It can help those with neuropathic pain, CRPS, and non-neuropathic pain conditions. The concept of administering a drug intermittently, with weeks between administration, using a drug with a relatively short half-life and exposing the patients to short-term side effects only after administration has attraction when compared to the day-in, day-out dosing, and hence side effects, associated with oral drug use.

Clonidine's effect in reducing opioid withdrawal reactions

There has been a very marked increase in the use of strong opioid medication in the treatment of chronic pain. Even when strong opioids are not used, many patients take codeine-based analgesics on a long-term basis as a pain-relieving strategy. Ultimately, many patients develop tolerance to the effects of these opioids. Should a patient wish to reduce and ultimately discontinue opioid use, then an opioid withdrawal reaction may be precipitated. Among the features of such a reaction are an increase in pain, anorexia, palpitations, insomnia, agitation, and sweating. These reactions can be highly unpleasant and can last for over one week. In monkeys treated with increasing doses of morphine to induce opioid dependence, withdrawal precipitates a withdrawal reaction which can be reduced by continuous clonidine administration. In humans, systemic clonidine appears to have the same effect.

Tizanadine

Tizanadine is marketed for the treatment of muscle spasm associated with multiple sclerosis but since it has an α-adrenoreceptor agonist effect one would expect it also to have analgesic properties. This supposition is backed up, to a certain extent, by study and case report evidence.

As would be expected with a drug active on α-adrenoreceptors, tizanadine can cause hypotension, dry mouth, and sedation. Indeed, in clinical practice this sedation can be utilized to aid sleep by giving the greater proportion of the proposed dose at night. The hypotension associated with both tizanadine and clonidine is of approximately equal proportions. Practically this offers some advantage to the intermittent epidural injection of clonidine over the daily dosing required with tizanadine as troublesome hypotension would then also be only intermittent as opposed to day-in, day-out.

Tizanadine has been shown to have pain-relieving effects in the following conditions. For example:
• Tension headache
• Cluster headache
• Chronic daily headache
• Low back pain
• Neuropathic pain
• Refractory trigeminal neuralgia
• Myofascial pain

A further interesting finding with tizanadine use is its ability to reduce gastric irritation associated with non-steroidal anti-inflammatory use. This property emerged from a study where the effects of tizanadine were being compared to those of non-steroidal anti-inflammatories. Subjects receiving just the anti-inflammatory reported symptoms of gastric irritation significantly more frequent than those receiving the anti-inflammatory and tizanadine together.

Conclusions

Drugs active at α-adrenoreceptors offer some hope of producing pain relief. The clinical evidence defining their place in pain management is, as yet, light and largely anecdotal. Nevertheless, epidural use of clonidine can give prolonged relief in conditions otherwise resistant to "conventional" pain therapy, whereas oral tizanadine has a place in management particularly where there is a need for muscle relaxation and sedation as well.

Bibliography

Bhatnagar S, Mishra S, Madhurima S et al. Clonidine as an analgesic adjuvant to continuous paravertebral bupivicaine for post-thoracotomy pain. *Anaesth Intensive Care* 2006; 34: 586–91.

Casati A, Magistris L, Fanelli G et al. Small-dose clonidine prolongs postoperative analgesia after sciatic-femoral nerve blocks with 0.75% ropivicaine for foot surgery. *Anesth Analg* 2000; 91: 388–92.

Chen SQ, Zhai HF, Cui YY et al. Clonidine attenuates morphine withdrawal and subsequent drug sensitization in rhesus monkeys. *Acta Pharmacol Sin* 2007; 28: 473–83.

Cucchiaro G, Ganesh A. The effects of clonidine on postoperative analgesia after peripheral nerve blockade in children. *Anesth Analg* 2007; 104: 532–7.

Fogelholm R, Murros K. Tizanadine in chronic tension-type headache: a placebo controlled double-blind cross-over study. *Headache* 1992; 32: 509–13.

Huang YS, Lin LC, Huh BK et al. Epidural clonidine for postoperative pain after total knee arthroplasty: a dose-response study. *Anesth Analg* 2007; 104: 1230–5.

Hutschala D, Mascher H, Schmetterer L et al. Clonidine added to bupivicaine enhances and prolongs analgesia after brachial plexus block via a local mechanism in healthy volunteers. *Eur J Anaesthesiol* 2004; 21: 198–204.

Malanga GA, Gwynn MW, Smith R, Miller D. Tizanadine is effective in the treatment of myofascial pain syndrome. *Pain Physician* 2002; 5: 422–32.

Memis D, Turan A, Karamanlioglu B et al. The effect of tramadol or clonidine added to intraperitoneal bupivicaine on postoperative pain in total abdominal hysterectomy. *J Opioid Manag* 2005; 1: 77–82.

Parker RK, Connelly NR, Lucas T et al. Epidural clonidine added to a bupivicaine infusion increases analgesic duration in labor without adverse maternal or fetal effects. *J Anesth* 2007; 21: 142–7.

Pratap JN, Shankar RK, Goroszeniuk T. Co-injection of clonidine prolongs the anesthetic effect of lidocaine skin infiltration by a peripheral action. *Anesth Analg* 2007; 104: 982–3.

Romero-Sandoval A, Bynum T, Eisenach JC. Analgesia induced by perineural clonidine is enhanced in persistent neuritis. *Neuroreport* 2007; 18: 67–71.

Romero-Sandoval A, Eisenach JC. Perineural clonidine reduces mechanical hypersensitivity and cytokine production in established nerve injury. *Anesthesiology* 2006; 104: 351–5.

Sirdalud Ternelin Asia-Pacific Study Group. Efficacy and gastro protective effects of tizanadine plus diclofenac versus placebo plus diclofenac in patients with painful muscle spasms. *Curr Ther Res* 1998; 59: 13–22.

CHAPTER 10
Lamotrigine

It is now established beyond doubt that anti-epileptic drugs (AEDs) can reduce pain and in particular that of a neuropathic type. This effect is shared by most members of the class. The AEDs are a group of drugs that are unified by their clinical effect, namely, their ability to reduce seizures rather than by a common mode of action. Therefore, if one member of the group fails to reduce pain, or causes unacceptable side effects, then there may be logic in trying a different member of the group.

Currently just three of the AEDs have a specific pain indication. Carbamazepine is indicated for trigeminal neuralgia with gabapentin having a US licence for postherpetic neuralgia (neuropathic pain in the UK) and pregabalin for fibromyalgia, postherpetic neuralgia and painful diabetic neuropathy (peripheral neuropathic pain in the UK). The gulf between what is officially licensed and what can be effective is as wide among the AEDs as any other drug group. The possession of a marketing authorization or specific indication does not suggest that a particular drug is superior than any other drug which may be used "off-label." It merely suggests that evidence of efficacy has been sought and presented in an acceptable way to the licensing authorities. From a purely scientific perspective, we lack the comparative studies that would advise us as to the best drug choices in an individual drug class.

Side effects of anti-epileptic drugs

When we consider drug side effects, much of the available evidence comes from drug studies which are almost universally of short duration. Therefore side effects recorded are the acute side effects and not those associated with long-term therapy. Since neuropathic pain, the primary indication for AED use is often long term if not lifelong, consideration should be given not only to the acute side effects associated with the use of a particular drug, but also to the long-term consequences of its use.

Pain Management: Expanding the Pharmacological Options, Gary J. McCleane. © 2008
Blackwell Publishing, ISBN: 978-1-4051-7823-5.

When the AEDs are compared in terms of propensity to alter body weight, Biton (2003) found that carbamazepine and valproate increase weight, topiramate and felbamate decrease it while lamotrigine, levetiracetam, and phenytoin are weight neutral.

In terms of their effect on cognition, as with much of the data on other potential side effects, it is based on work done largely in subjects with epilepsy. Given that epilepsy may itself cause CNS abnormalities due both to the underlying cause of the epilepsy and to the effect of previous seizures, the interpretation of this data is problematical. That said, it can give some insight into the possible CNS side effects in patients with, for example, neuropathic pain. Aldenkamp and colleagues (2003) suggest that oxcarbazepine and lamotrigine do not affect cognitive function in either healthy volunteers or epilepsy patients, while Hirsch and colleagues (2003) suggest that sodium valproate produces few cognitive side effects.

Martin and colleagues (1999) examined the possible effects on cognitive function produced by topiramate, gabapentin, and lamotrigine in healthy young volunteers. They found that topiramate did have an effect on cognitive function while lamotrigine and gabapentin had little effect. The finding that lamotrigine and gabapentin have little effect on cognitive function is confirmed in a review by Goldberg and Burdick (2001). Aldenkamp (2001) compared phenytoin, carbamazepine, and sodium valproate. The cognitive impairment produced by phenytoin was greater than that produced by carbamazepine or sodium valproate.

Besag (2004) has reviewed the data pertaining to the behavioral side effects of nine of the more recently introduced AEDs. Vigabatrin and topiramate have been associated with both psychosis and depression. He suggests that lamotrigine is largely associated with improvement rather than deterioration in mood and behavior while gabapentin has relatively little effect on behavior. The data on tiagabine and oxcarbazepine is too limited to allow useful interpretation.

Overall, after the review of the literature, LaRoche and Helmers (2004) have stated that the more recently introduced AEDs have overall a better tolerability than the older members of this class (Table 10.1).

Therefore, from a side effect perspective, lamotrigine may expose the patient to a lessened risk of troublesome side effects when compared to other AEDs. In particular, the lack of weight gain and minimal risk of sedation contrast it to other widely prescribed AEDs and make it a more attractive option for long-term therapy than many others in the class. In my own practice, lamotrigine is the first choice AED.

Perhaps the most prominent side effect associated with lamotrigine use is skin rash. There is even an isolated case report of a fatal onset of Stephens Johnson syndrome with lamotrigine use. The risk of skin rash is increased by rapid dose escalation. And so achievement of a potentially

Table 10.1 Side effects of anti-epileptic drugs.

Side effect	Anti-epileptics in general	Lamotrigine
Weight	Weight gain	Weight neutral
Sedation	Sedative	Non-sedative
Cognition	Cognitive impairment	No effect
Teratogenesis	Risk with some, others not established	Probably little risk

therapeutic dose may take many weeks with that relatively long delay before any beneficial effect may be apparent.

Mode of action

Lamotrigine has an effect on voltage-gated cation channels and on glutamate release. Carbamazepine, oxcarbazepine, and phenytoin also have actions on neuronal sodium channels while it is thought that gabapentin and pregabalin interact with the α-δ2 sub-unit of the calcium channel, clonazepam on gamma amino butyric acid (GABA) mediated transmission while lacosamide has its actions on strychnine-sensitive glycine channels. Although lamotrigine, carbamazepine, oxcarbazepine, and phenytoin all have actions on sodium channels, from a clinical perspective one can have an analgesic effect in a given patient while another has no effect. This may be because they interact with different sodium channels.

Clinical use of lamotrigine

Undoubtedly there are fewer pain studies on lamotrigine than there are with gabapentin or pregabalin. Of course, since the manufacturers of lamotrigine did not pursue a product licence for lamotrigine in the treatment of neuropathic pain, they sponsored fewer studies, and none of the size that were undertaken with gabapentin or pregabalin.

That said, controlled trials have confirmed a pain-relieving effect in the following conditions:
- Painful diabetic neuropathy
- HIV-associated painful sensory neuropathy
- Neuralgia after nerve section
- Spinal cord injury pain
- Central poststroke pain
- Trigeminal neuralgia
- Postoperative pain

Case report evidence also suggests that it can reduce the neuropathic pain associated with multiple sclerosis and complex regional pain syndrome

(CRPS) type 1. In the latter case the burning pain, allodynia and intermittent swelling, and discoloration all associated with the condition were lessened by lamotrigine treatment.

It could be argued that if there is controlled trial evidence to suggest a pain-relieving effect of lamotrigine in at least six neuropathic pain syndromes then it is likely that this effect is replicated in many other conditions where neuropathic pain is evident.

However, not all studies have shown a positive effect with lamotrigine use. This may be partially due to inadequate doses being administered. In a study of 100 patients with neuropathic pain of mixed etiology, I found that 200 mg daily of lamotrigine had no analgesic effect (McCleane, 1999). It does seem that a dose of at least 300 mg daily is required for pain relief to be produced. Despite the negative findings of this study, it should be emphasized that lamotrigine remains my first choice AED, albeit at a dose higher than that utilized in the study.

In one study of the effect of lamotrigine on patients with intractable sciatica, the authors found that there was a direct correlation between the plasma concentration of lamotrigine and the mean weekly spontaneous pain scores (Eisenberg and colleagues, 2003). It has been suggested that the serum level of lamotrigine can be influenced by concomitant drug consumption with these drugs being metabolized at a similar cytochrome P450 site to lamotrigine. It would not be unreasonable to assume that such influences would affect the dose of lamotrigine needed to achieve pain relief.

A single comparative study has been reported in patients with painful diabetic neuropathy. The subjects were treated with lamotrigine in a dose of up to 100 mg twice daily or with amitriptyline at a dose of up to 50 mg at night. Pain relief was comparable in both groups, but significantly more side effects, and in particular sedation (43% of those treated) with amitriptyline. The authors concluded that lamotrigine could be perceived as the first-line treatment of painful diabetic neuropathy, ahead of amitriptyline, not on the basis of efficacy but rather because of its greater tolerability. Given that other studies have shown that doses in excess of 200 mg daily are required to achieve useful pain relief, one wonders what the results of this study may have looked like had a higher dose of lamotrigine been used.

Clinical use of lamotrigine

The following guidelines on the use of lamotrigine represent the fashion in which we have used this drug in clinical practice in over 12 years of use:

1 Consideration is given to lamotrigine use when the symptoms and signs of neuropathic pain are present (paresthesia/dyesthesia, shooting/lancinating pain, burning pain, allodynia, hyperesthesia).

2 Where possible lamotrigine is used in place of, rather than in addition to, other pain medication: if this other pain medication was working satisfactorily then consideration of lamotrigine use in the first place would be unnecessary.

3 Lamotrigine is commenced at a dose of 50 mg daily and increased by 50 mg each week until a 300 mg daily dose is achieved after 6 weeks.

4 If satisfactory pain relief is apparent at a lower dose, then escalation to the 300 mg dose is halted at the effective dose.

5 When 300 mg daily dose is achieved, the patient remains on this dose for 1 week. If after that period satisfactory relief is not apparent, then it is discontinued.

6 The dose of lamotrigine can be administered in divided or a single daily dose (the half-life of lamotrigine is just over 30 h).

7 After prolonged successful use, the patient may try to see if they can do without the lamotrigine. In this situation they should reduce the lamotrigine by 50 mg daily per week and cease dose decrease if pain returns. It is necessary to decrease the dose slowly because of the long half-life of the drug.

8 Should lamotrigine be stopped and pain return, for some reason it is not unusual for subsequent lamotrigine use to be ineffective.

Conclusions

Despite the increasing number of anti-epileptics available, to date only three are licensed for use in patients with neuropathic pain. Of the available drugs in this class, lamotrigine has a number of distinct advantages in terms of long-term tolerability and effectiveness that dictate that it is a drug that should be considered in any patient with neuropathic pain. Indeed, in my opinion, it remains the most effective and most easily tolerated of all available AEDs. That said, it is not universally effective and there remains logic in a trial of an alternate anti-epileptic should lamotrigine therapy at a suitable dose be ineffective.

Bibliography

Aldenkamp AP. Effects of antiepileptic drugs on cognition. *Epilepsia* 2001; 42 (Suppl): 46–9.

Aldenkamp AP, De Krom M, Reijs R. Newer antiepileptic drugs and cognitive issues. *Epilepsia* 2003; 44 (Suppl): 21–29.

Besag FM. Behavioural effects of the newer antiepileptic drugs: an update. *Expert Opin Drug Saf* 2004; 3: 1–8.

Bonicalzi V, Canavero S, Cerutti F et al. Lamotrigine reduces total postoperative analgesic requirement: a randomized double-blind, placebo-controlled pilot study. *Surgery* 1997; 122: 567–70.

Biton V. Effect of antiepileptic drugs on bodyweight: overview and clinical implications for the treatment of epilepsy. *CNS Drugs* 2003; 17: 781–91.

Devulder J. The relevance of monitoring lamotrigine serum concentrations in chronic pain patients. *Acta Neurol Belg* 2006; 106: 15–18.

Eisenberg E, Damunni G, Hoffer E et al. Lamotrigine for intractable sciatica: correlation between dose, plasma concentration and analgesia. *Eur J Pain* 2003; 7: 485–91.

Eisenberg E, Lurie Y, Braker C et al. Lamotrigine reduces painful diabetic neuropathy: a randomized, controlled study. *Neurology* 2001; 57: 505–9.

Finnerup NB, Sindrup SH, Bach FW et al. Lamotrigine in spinal cord injury pain: a randomized controlled trial. *Pain* 2002; 96: 375–63.

Goldberg JF, Burdick KE. Cognitive side effects of anticonvulsants. *J Clin Psychiatry* 2001; 62 (Suppl): 27–33.

Hirsch E, Schmitz B, Carreno M. Epilepsy, antiepileptic drugs (AEDs) and cognition. *Acta Neurol Scand Suppl* 2003; 108: 23–32.

Jose VM, Bhansali A, Hota D, Pandhi P. Randomized double-blind study comparing the efficacy and safety of lamotrigine and amitriptyline in painful diabetic neuropathy. *Diabet Med* 2007; 24: 377–83.

LaRoche SM, Helmers SL. The new antiepileptic drugs: scientific review. *JAMA* 2004; 291: 605–14.

Martin R, Kuzniecky R, Ho S et al. Cognitive effects of Topiramate, gabapentin, and lamotrigine in healthy young adults. *Neurology* 1999; 52: 321–7.

McCleane GJ. 200 mg lamotrigine has no analgesic effect in neuropathic pain: a randomised, double-blind placebo controlled trial. *Pain* 1999; 83: 105–7.

McCleane GJ. The symptoms of complex regional pain syndrome type 1 alleviated with lamotrigine: a report of 8 cases. *Clin J Pain* 2000; 16; 171–3.

McCleane GJ. Lamotrigine in the management of neuropathic pain: a review of the literature. *Clin J Pain* 2000; 16: 321–6.

Sandner-Kiesling A, Rumpold-Seitlinger G, Dorn C et al. Lamotrigine monotherapy for control of neuralgia after nerve section. *Acta Anaesthesiol Scand* 2002; 46: 1261–4.

Simpson DM, McArthur JC, Olney R et al. Lamotrigine for HIV-associated painful sensory neuropathies: a placebo-controlled trial. *Neurology* 2003; 60: 1508–14.

Simpson DM, Olney R, McArthur JC et al. A placebo-controlled trial of lamotrigine for painful HIV-associated neuropathy. *Neurology* 2000; 54: 2115–19.

Vestergaard K, Andersen G, Gottrup H et al. Lamotrigine for central poststroke pain: a randomized controlled trial. *Neurology* 2001; 56: 184–90.

Vink AI, Tuchman M, Safirstein B et al. Lamotrigine for treatment of pain associated with diabetic neuropathy: results of two randomized, double-blind, placebo-controlled studies. *Pain* 2007; 128: 169–79.

Zakrzewska JM, Chaudhry Z, Nurmikko TJ et al. Lamotrigine (Lamictal) in refractory trigeminal neuralgia: results from a double-blind placebo controlled crossover trial. *Pain* 1997; 73: 223–30.

CHAPTER 11

5HT$_3$ Antagonists

Most practitioners will have experience in using 5HT$_3$ antagonists in the management of postoperative nausea and vomiting and in the prophylaxis and treatment of nausea and vomiting associated with cancer chemotherapy. Fewer will be aware of the body of scientific and clinical evidence that suggests that they can also have useful pain-relieving effects as well. That evidence suggests, with varying levels of supportive data, that 5HT$_3$ antagonists can or may, have the following effects:

- They can reduce neuropathic pain.
- They can reduce the pain associated with fibromyalgia.
- They can reduce the symptoms of irritable bowel syndrome.
- They can reduce localized pain when given by local tender spot injection.
- They can reduce the pain caused by injection of irritant substances.
- They can reduce metastatic bone pain.
- They might have an effect on opioid tolerance.

The 5HT$_3$ antagonists

This group of compounds have been available for clinical use for over 10 years and individual members of the class differ in their pharmacokinetic properties. They are available in a variety of formulations (Table 11.1).

Neuropathic pain

Neurokinin-1 expressing neurons (NK-1) are situated in the superficial lamina of the spinal dorsal horn, utilize substance P as a neurotransmitter and are responsible for relaying a peripheral nociceptive stimulus to the parabrachial area and hence to the cerebrum. This causes a descending signal to the periaqueductal gray area and hence to the rostroventral medulla causing

Pain Management: Expanding the Pharmacological Options, Gary J. McCleane. © 2008
Blackwell Publishing, ISBN: 978-1-4051-7823-5.

Table 11.1 Formulation

5HT₃ antagonist	Tablet	Syrup	Lyophilisate	Suppository	Injection
Alosetron	X				
Dolasetron	X				X
Granisetron	X				X
Ondansetron	X	X	X	X	X
Palonestron					X
Tropisetron	X				X

activation of descending serotinergic and noradrenergic drives on the spinal dorsal horn which inhibit further spino-cerebral nociceptive signaling.

Experimentally, the function of the NK-1 expressing neurons can be terminated by application of the specific toxin substance P – saponin conjugate. When this is done in animals that have formalin applied to their paws, the second phase of the so-called formalin response is significantly reduced. In this response there is normally an acute nociceptive response (the so-called first phase response) followed by a slower and more prolonged nociceptive response (the second phase) which can be measured behaviorally by counting, for example, the licking activity by the animal of its paw, or electrophysiologically by measuring the electrical activity in deep dorsal horn cells. Therefore, ablation of NK-1 expressing neurones has an antinociceptive effect, at least with this experimental model. This is reinforced by the fact that in animals bred with genetic absence of NK-1 neurons a similar reduction in the second phase of the formalin response occurs.

In contrast, when a carrageenan model of inflammation is used, depletion of these neurons has no effect suggesting that the role of NK-1 expressing neurons is dependent on the nociceptive stimulus.

When the behavioral or electrophysiological measurements are repeated in animals having formalin application to paws and this time the 5HT₃ antagonist ondansetron is applied spinally, an exactly similar reduction in the second phase of the formalin response occurs as when substance P – saponin conjugate is applied. This implies two things:

1 That 5HT₃ antagonists may have an analgesic effect.
2 If application of a 5HT₃ antagonist reduces spino-cerebral nociceptive signaling when we know that 5HT₃ agonists normally have this effect, then it suggests that as well as the well-known bulbo-spinal serotinergic inhibitory pathways there may also be descending serotinergic facilitatory pathways as well.

Clinically it has been shown that a single injection of ondansetron in humans with neuropathic pain resistant to previous pharmacological therapy reduces that neuropathic pain. No longer-term dosing studies nor studies where oral ondansetron or other 5HT₃ antagonists are used have been carried out.

Therefore, there is suggestion that clinically ondansetron may reduce neuropathic pain and that there is a logical explanation for why that may occur. Clearly significant work needs to be done to verify this observation. From an entirely practical perspective, ondansetron could be given parenterally in patients with acute flare-ups of neuropathic pain or to those in whom the oral route is unavailable. The major drawbacks of treatment are that at present, all 5HT$_3$ antagonists are extremely expensive, to the extent that they probably could not be used in a day-in, day-out basis but may be a useful treatment during a period of flare-up of neuropathic pain. The two major side effects of continued 5HT$_3$ use are headache and constipation.

Fibromyalgia

A number of studies suggest that the 5HT$_3$ antagonist tropisetron, given either orally or intravenously, can reduce the pain associated with fibromyalgia and improve patient quality of life. Given the well-known difficulties in treating this condition, anything with as low a risk of producing side effects as tropisetron should be of considerable interest. Work remains to be done to investigate the effect of the other 5HT$_3$ antagonists to see if they replicate the pain-relieving effect of tropisetron.

In an intriguing aside, it is universally acknowledged that the tricyclic antidepressants can reduce neuropathic pain and that of fibromyalgia. At least some of this effect is mediated by their effects on augmenting the descending bulbo-spinal serotinergic inhibitory drives. It has been shown in animal models that amitriptyline dosing of rats with neuropathic pain caused by spinal nerve ligation reduces the allodynia in the paw on the side of injury. But when these animals are treated with amitriptyline, the paw on the contralateral side to the injury becomes hyperesthetic, where previously they were normal after commencement of the amitriptyline! Could this be because it augments the descending bulbo-spinal facilitatory drive in the absence of spino-cerebral nociceptive signaling? If so, logic would suggest that co-administration of a 5HT$_3$ antagonist could ablate this response, but work on the potential augmentative effect of a 5HT$_3$ antagonist on tricyclic antidepressants remains to be done.

Irritable bowel syndrome

This chronic disabling condition is not infrequently associated with fibromyalgia. The 5HT$_3$ antagonist alosetron currently holds a product licence in the US for use in females with diarrhea preponderant irritable bowel syndrome. This restrictive label is because this was the group who responded to treatment in the proving studies with others having a less marked or absent response. When alosetron is used, the number of bowel motions passed decrease and with this pain relief increases. However, use is not without dangers. There have been case reports of alosetron treatment leading to ischemic colitis.

Not only have $5HT_3$ antagonist been shown to help some with irritable bowel syndrome but also to reduce the behavioral responses to noxious colorectal distension in animal models. The effect of other $5HT_3$ antagonists on irritable bowel syndrome remains to be defined. Anecdotal evidence does suggest that indeed other $5HT_3$ antagonists do have this property.

Alosetron does not have a marketing authorization in the UK.

Local tender spot injection

Injection of local anesthetic and corticosteroid is a common procedure in pain and rheumatological practice. This can be into a tender muscle, inflamed joint, tendon, ligament, or bursa, for example. Use of these drugs in this fashion is tried and tested, but not without real and potential drawbacks. Lipoatrophy and the creation of localized telangectasia are not uncommon in the short term, while the worry of tendon weakening or osteoporosis inhibits repeated treatment. This can be most frustrating as these injections are often particularly effective. Clinical reports and experience suggest that use of a $5HT_3$ antagonist in place of a corticosteroid can be rewarded by pain relief of a similar magnitude and duration, but devoid of the short- and long-term potential risks of corticosteroid injection. For example, in clinical practice Achilles tendinitis can be a very troubling condition. A significant worry associated with corticosteroid injection would be tendon weakening which may result in tendon rupture. Injection of $5HT_3$ antagonist can give pain relief with no risk of rupture.

When used clinically for localized injection, it is not unusual for $5HT_3$ antagonists to cause a localized pain flare, which may last several days, before relief is apparent. As with corticosteroid injection, it is usual to co-inject a local anesthetic, but whether this has any influence on the time to onset and ultimate duration of pain relief is questionable.

It seems that $5HT_3$ antagonists can also have the same action on the duration of effect of a nerve block as a corticosteroid and can be used as an alternative to corticosteroids for this reason.

Pain caused by injection of irritant substances

Those involved in anesthesiological practice in particular will know that injection of certain drugs is associated with pain, which may at times be severe. A number of strategies exist for reducing this pain, one of which is injection of a 5HT$_3$ antagonist prior to injection of the irritating substance such as the IV induction agent propofol. Given that 5HT$_3$ antagonists are commonly given during an anesthetic to reduce postoperative nausea and vomiting, it would be a simple task to pre-treat the patient with the 5HT$_3$ antagonist rather than defer its use until later in the procedure in the hope that it could act as an antiemetic and also reduce injection-related pain.

One suggestion for the mechanism by which ondansetron reduces pain of injection is that it has sodium channel blocking effects. Alternatively, ondansetron could reduce pain by its effect on peripheral 5HT$_3$ receptors. These are thought to be involved in inflammatory pain, hyperalgesia, and vasodilation around a site of inflammation.

Metastatic bone pain

A single animal study suggests that ondansetron can reduce metastatic bone pain. This has not been verified in humans, nor has the effect been confirmed when other 5HT$_3$ antagonists are used. It does emphasize, however, that there is no suggestion that 5HT$_3$ antagonists are universally effective for all types of pain, but rather that they can have an effect in certain defined conditions.

Opioid tolerance

In an animal model, tolerance to the antinociceptive effects of strong opioids is remarkably easy to induce. The issue of tolerance to opioids in human clinical practice is much more contentious. In animal models, administration of opioids causes changes in the activity of NK-1 expressing neurons in the superficial lamina of the dorsal horn which leads to a need to increase opioid dose to achieve the same antinociceptive effect. When morphine is administered to rats, the expression of substance P and NK-1 receptors in the spinal dorsal horn is increased and the release of substance P evoked by capsaicin administration is also increased. The NK-1 expressing neurons subsume a paradoxical pronociceptive function which is reversed by administration of NK-1 receptor antagonists.

Subsequent studies have shown that co-administration of the 5HT$_3$ antagonist ondansetron prevents the onset of this antinociceptive tolerance. Again, the issue of whether this effect is replicated in humans has not, as yet, been clarified.

Clinical use of 5HT$_3$ antagonists

While 5HT$_3$ antagonists may ultimately find a place in the management of metastatic bone pain and in reducing opioid tolerance at present this use would be speculative. Their use in the other circumstances mentioned above is more firmly based. From a practical perspective the following guidelines for use is suggested and are based on my own personal experience of use of these drugs.

Neuropathic pain

Use of a 5HT$_3$ antagonist in the treatment of neuropathic pain may be reserved for management of a flare-up in view of the considerable cost if more long-term therapy were instituted and the risk of severe constipation. Ondansetron 8 mg intravenously or orally (either as a tablet or the lyophilisate) can be used, repeated up to three times a day.

Fibromyalgia

Again 5HT$_3$ antagonists may be reserved for treatment of a flare-up although they can be used on a more long-term basis if the patient also has diarrhea-preponderant irritable bowel syndrome. Again, ondansetron 8 mg intravenously or orally can be used three times daily.

Tender point injections, intra-articular, and nerve blocks

In all of these procedures a local anesthetic is co-administered with the 5HT$_3$ antagonist. Since injection of 5HT$_3$ antagonists can cause pain before they cause pain relief, and because this pain flare can last for up to several days, if a local anesthetic is used it may be preferable to use a long-acting local anesthetic such as bupivicaine. Granisetron 2 mg can be given with the local anesthetic regardless of whether it is being used for a tender spot injection, injected into a joint or if it is being used for a nerve block.

It is suggested that ondansetron be used for neuropathic pain and fibromyalgia treatment and granisetron for tender point, intra-articular, and nerve block injections. There is no logic to why a differing 5HT$_3$ antagonist is used in these circumstances and why other 5HT$_3$ antagonists are not used. It merely reflects habit.

Conclusions

The 5HT$_3$ antagonists are a freely available group of drugs that have a long pedigree in the treatment of postoperative and chemotherapy-related nausea and vomiting. They can also reduce neuropathic pain and that related to fibromyalgia along with regularizing the bowel pattern and reducing pain in some patients with irritable bowel syndrome. In addition to these effects, it seems that 5HT₃ antagonists can also replace the use of corticosteroids when tender spot injection, intra-articular injection, or nerve blocks, for example, are being considered.

At least some of the pain-relieving effects of the 5HT₃ antagonists may be related to their effect of reducing the activity of NK-1 expressing neurons that are primarily located in the superficial laminae of the spinal dorsal horn cells.

Side effects associated with 5HT₃ use include headache and constipation, but perhaps the greatest impediment to their more widespread use is their considerable expense. However, they are commendable because of their low risk of causing serious side effects and because many practitioners will be comfortable with their use as they will have experience with administering them as antiemetics.

Bibliography

Ambesh SP, Dubey PK, Sinha PK. Ondansetron pre-treatment to alleviate pain on propofol injection: a randomized, controlled, double-blind study. *Anesth Analg* 1999; 89: 197–9.

Esser MJ, Chase T, Allen GV, Sawynok J. Chronic administration of amitriptyline and caffeine in a rat model of neuropathic pain: multiple interactions. *Eur J Pharmacol* 2001; 430: 211–18.

Esser MJ, Sawynok J. Acute amitriptyline in a rat model of neuropathic pain: differential symptom and route effects. *Pain* 1999; 80: 643–53.

Giordano J, Daleo C, Sacks SM. Topical ondansetron attenuates nociceptive and inflammatory effects of intradermal capsaicin in humans. *Eur J Pharmacol* 1998; 13–4.

King T, Gardell LR, Wang R et al. Role of NK-1 neurotransmission in opioid-induced hyperalgesia. *Pain* 2005; 116; 276–88.

McCleane GJ. Tricyclic antidepressants, SSRIs and descending serotinergic facilitatory pathways: could 5HT₃ antagonists prevent paradoxical pain? A hypothesis. *J Neuropathic Pain Symptom Palliation* 2006; 1: 57–60.

McCleane GJ, Suzuki R, Dickenson AH. Does a single IV injection of the 5HT₃ receptor antagonist ondansetron have an analgesic effect in neuropathic pain? A double-blind, placebo-controlled cross-over study. *Anesth Analg* 2003; 97: 1474–8.

Miranda A, Peles S, McLean PG, Sengupta JN. Effects of the 5HT₃ receptor antagonist, alosetron, in a rat model of somatic and visceral hyperalgesia. *Pain* 2006; 126: 54–63.

Muller W, Fiebich BL, Stratz T. New treatment options using 5HT₃ receptor antagonists in rheumatic diseases. *Curr Top Med Chem* 2006; 6: 2035–42.

Muller W, Stratz T. Local treatment of tendinopathies and myofascial pain syndromes with the 5HT₃ receptor antagonist tropisetron. *Scand J Rheumatol Suppl* 2004; 119: 44–8.

Rahman W, Suzuki R, Rygh LJ, Dickenson AH. Descending serotinergic facilitation mediated through rat spinal 5HT₃ receptors is unaltered following carrageenan inflammation. *Neurosci Lett* 2004; 361: 229–32.

Samborski W, Stratz T, Mackiewicz S, Muller W. Intra-articular treatment of arthritides and activated osteoarthritis with the 5HT$_3$ receptor antagonist tropisetron. A double-blind study compared with methylprednisolone. *Scand J Rheumatol Suppl* 2004; 119: 51–4.

Stratz T, Farber L, Varga B et al. Fibromyalgia treatment with intravenous tropisetron. *Drugs Exp Clin Res* 2001; 27: 113–18.

Tolk J, Kohnen R, Muller W. Intravenous treatment of fibromyalgia with the 5HT$_3$ receptor antagonist tropisetron in a rheumatological practice. *Scand J Rheumatol Suppl* 2004; 119: 72–5.

Vera-Portocarrero LP, Zhang ET, King T et al. Spinal NK-1 receptor expressing neurons mediate opioid-induced hyperalgesia and antinociceptive tolerance via activation of descending pathways. *Pain* 2007; 129: 35–45.

Ye JH, Mui WC, Ren J et al. Ondansetron exhibits the properties of a local anesthetic. *Anesth Analg* 1997; 85: 1116–21.

CHAPTER 12

Cholecystokinin Antagonists

Despite the almost universal use of opioids in all fields of pain management, this class of drugs are associated with well-defined issues which include partial efficacy in some pain conditions and analgesic tolerance with sustained use. Other complications of use may be, at least to a certain extent, dose related. Therefore, if it were possible to maximize analgesic potential from an opioid, minimize the dose required to achieve pain relief and reduce the need to escalate dose as tolerance occurs then this would be of great help. It may be that the cholecystokinin (CCK) antagonists represent one strategy in achieving this aim.

Cholecystokinin

The peptide CCK was initially attributed with a role in gallbladder secretion by Ivy and Goldberg back in 1928. It was observed that when blood was taken from dogs after feeding and given to other dogs, their gallbladders contracted, suggesting that feeding caused release of a hormonal substance that was active on the gallbladder.

When foods containing fatty and amino acids are ingested and pass along with endogenously secreted hydrochloric acid into the duodenum they cause CCK release which leads to gallbladder contraction, pancreatic exocrine secretion along with pyloric contraction, and gastric relaxation. The expulsion of bile acids into the small bowel causes a reflex suppression of further CCK release.

There the story rested until the mid-1970s when it was realized that CCK also existed in the central nervous system and that its function there was not related to the gastrointestinal tract. Since there were differences in the structure and function of the CCK found in the gut and the central nervous system they were given different titles. Therefore the CCK found in the gut was labeled as "CCK A" (where A refers to alimentary) and "CCK B" (where the B refers to brain).

Pain Management: Expanding the Pharmacological Options, Gary J. McCleane. © 2008 Blackwell Publishing, ISBN: 978-1-4051-7823-5.

Role of cholecystokinin in the nervous system

Cholecystokinin appears to subserve many functions in the central nervous system with its actions being complex and diffuse. They can be summarized as including the following effects:
- An action on norepinephrine in the supraoptic nucleus.
- It facilitates the antianalgesic effect of dynorphin.
- It inhibits opioid binding to μ and κ opioid receptors.
- It reverses the μ and κ opioid suppression of increase in the free intracellular Ca^{2+} following K^+ depolarization.
- It modulates dopamine release from the nucleus acumbens.
- It inhibits *OFF* cells in the rostral ventral medulla.
- It decreases α_2-adrenergic-mediated antinociception.
- It inhibits release of [Leu^5] enkephalin.

A number of factors influence the levels of free CCK and of mRNA for CCK in the central nervous system. Critical among these are neural injury and opioid consumption. Both of these increase central nervous system CCK. It has been shown that in animals with surgically inflicted neural injury that the levels of free CCK are equal in sham-operated animals and those with neural injury but who do not display the signs of neuropathic pain. In those injured animals with signs of neuropathic pain the levels of CCK are markedly increased.

Cholecystokinin as an anti-opioid peptide

When an opioid is administered, in a variety of animal pain models a well-known antinociceptive effect is apparent. This effect is the basis of our use of opioids as analgesics. However, when CCK is administered along with the opioid, a lesser or no antinociceptive effect is observed. If the nociceptive test is applied, opioid administered to produce an antinociceptive effect and then CCK is administered, then the opioid-induced antinociceptive effect is abolished. It therefore seems that CCK acts as an opioid peptide.

Cholecystokinin antagonists

One of the first CCK antagonists to be produced was the mixed CCK A and B antagonist proglumide. This has relatively weak receptor affinity but does also seem to possess inherent δ opioid agonist effects. It was originally produced for the treatment of peptic ulcer disease until the H_2 antagonists became available and were seen to be more effective in this

Table 12.1 Cholecystokinin antagonists.

A antagonists	B antagonists	Mixed A and B antagonists
L364,718	L365,260	Proglumide
Loxiglumide	YM022	
TO632	PD135,158	
FK480	PD134,308	
Asperlicin	L740,093	
Lorglumide	L365,031	
PD135,666	LY262,691	
	RP73870	
	YF476	

indication. As previously mentioned, CCK antagonists may be of the A, B, or mixed A and B varieties (Table 12.1).

Effect of CCK antagonists on opioid-derived antinociception

One of the first reports of a CCK antagonist enhancing the antinociceptive effect of an opioid dates from as far back as 1985 when it was shown that proglumide, when given systemically, intrathecally or intracerebrally enhanced morphine-derived antinociception in a rat radiant heat model. Further confirmation of this effect has been obtained in numerous studies. For example, in one intracerebroventricular injection of CCK-8 antagonized the antinociceptive effect of morphine in a mouse tail flick test. This effect is blocked by the specific CCK B antagonist PD135,158 but not by the CCK A antagonist lorglumide.

The majority of the studies suggest that CCK B antagonists such as L365,260, PD135,308, and PD135,158 have the greatest enhancing effect on opioid-derived antinociception with others giving strong support for the mixed antagonist proglumide also having a strong effect. However, it should be noted that most, but not all, of the studies have been on rodent and murine models with an isolated report in a primate model suggesting that an A antagonist was more effective than a B antagonist. This finding is of great relevance for the human studies.

Effect of CCK antagonists on antinociceptive tolerance to opioids

Just as the evidence suggesting an opioid enhancing effect of CCK antagonists is not new, that suggesting an effect of CCK antagonists on opioid antinociceptive tolerance is also not new. As far back as 1984 it was shown that after only seven or eight subcutaneous injections of morphine in a rat model, antinociceptive tolerance was occurring. This effect was blocked by co-administration of proglumide. It is a recurring theme of many animal studies just how easily antinociceptive tolerance to opioids can be induced after a surprisingly short period of time and yet there is still debate in human practice about how real an issue analgesic tolerance actually is.

The consistent finding in animal studies is that CCK antagonists at least delay the onset and decrease the magnitude of antinociceptive tolerance.

Some insight into the possible central location at which tolerance is mediated is gained from the results of experiments where a cannula is inserted into the periaqueductal gray area of rats. Microinjections of morphine produce antinociception as quantified by tail flick or hot plate tests. When morphine microinjection is repeated twice daily, the antinociceptive effects disappear within 2 days. However, if each morphine microinjection is preceded by a microinjection of proglumide, the microinjection of morphine consistently produces an antinociceptive effect despite ongoing morphine treatment showing that tolerance is blocked. If the proglumide microinjections are suspended, subsequent morphine injections induce tolerance. In morphine tolerant rats, a single microinjection of proglumide is enough to restore the antinociceptive effects of morphine.

While the majority of animal studies examining opioid-induced antinociceptive tolerance use morphine as the opioid, one utilized the short-acting opioid alfentanil. Within 4 h of initiation of an alfentanil infusion in rats there is an approximately 95% reduction in initial antinociceptive effect of the alfentanil. When the CCK B antagonist L365,260 is co-administered, after 4 h there is a lesser decrease in antinociceptive effect to around 65% of initial levels. When proglumide is given with the alfentanil infusion, the reduction of initial antinociceptive effect is less again at 45% after 4 h.

Reversal of established tolerance

The majority of animal studies addressing the issue of antinociceptive tolerance with opioid use concentrate on prevention of tolerance. Several studies also look at the effect of CCK antagonists on established antinociceptive tolerance. They confirm that in animals with induced opioid antinociceptive tolerance, the addition of a CCK antagonist does in fact reverse the tolerance.

Despite the strong animal evidence that CCK antagonists can reduce opioid antinociceptive tolerance, there are absolutely no human studies examining this effect. Indeed the human pain literature as a whole is virtually devoid of studies looking at tolerance with any class of pain-relieving medication and yet tolerance is a real clinical issue.

Safety of CCK antagonists

If strong opioids are being used, particularly at higher doses, then there may be anxiety at adding a drug that magnifies the analgesic effect that opioid gives in case it also increases other opioid-related side effects, and particularly if it depresses respiration. A study in a primate model and human clinical studies reassure that addition of a CCK antagonist to a strong opioid may increase pain relief but does not cause respiratory depression.

If CCK antagonists do bring enhanced pain relief then they may allow opioid dose reduction and so could be associated, paradoxically, with a reduction in opioid-related side effects.

In practice, CCK antagonists themselves are remarkably devoid of serious side effects. The most commonly utilized, proglumide has an unpleasant taste and very occasionally causes a skin rash.

Human studies

While extensive animal evidence points to an opioid enhancing effect of CCK antagonists with an additional effect on antinociceptive tolerance, the human literature is slight and somewhat contradictory.

The suggested use of CCK antagonists, and in particular proglumide, is based on extensive clinical use, rather than on the weight of human scientific evidence.

A number of human studies have examined the effect of the mixed CCK A and B antagonist proglumide. They have shown that it enhances the analgesic effect of morphine and dihydrocodeine when being used to treat chronic neuropathic pain. Further studies show it to enhance the analgesic effect and duration action of morphine when used for third molar surgery. A single human study failed to find any opioid enhancing effect of proglumide when it was used in patients after major abdominal or gynaecological surgery. One issue from the human studies is that a great range of doses have been used from fractions of a milligram to 200 mg twice daily. Clearly proper dose finding studies are required to define the optimum dose of proglumide, particularly as there is some evidence with other CCK antagonists of a bell-shaped dose–response curve.

A further field where proglumide has been assessed is that of chronic pancreatitis. As most will know, this condition is noted for its resistance to analgesic treatment with an appearance that many patients seem to become addicted to opiates. It could be argued that they crave pain relief and since this is only partial with opioid use they ask for more opioid in the hope that this may increase relief. In a proportion of patients with chronic pancreatitis the levels of CCK are elevated and one would presume that these patients are at least partially resistant to opioid use. Clinically a proportion of patients with chronic pancreatitis derive useful and sustained relief from short-term infusion of proglumide.

The other CCK antagonist that has been studied in humans is the CCK B antagonist L365,260. A study in patients taking strong opioids for neuropathic pain failed to find any opioid enhancing effect. This is in contrast to the findings with the mixed A and B antagonist proglumide. However, there may be an explanation for this. We have seen of the strong and robust animal evidence that CCK antagonists enhance opioid-derived antinociception and attenuate antinociceptive tolerance. The animal literature suggests that the B antagonists have the greatest effect and yet a human study with a B antagonist has been negative. But almost all of the animal studies have been in rodent and murine models. A single study in a primate (monkey) model has shown that in this species the CCK A antagonist was the most efficacious. Perhaps the importance of either the A or B receptors is species dependent with the B receptor being important in mice and rats while the A receptor is of more importance in monkeys and humans.

The CCK A antagonist loxiglumide has been examined in patients with biliary colic and compared to conventional treatment with the anticholinergic hyoscine. It has been shown that the loxiglumide was significantly more effective at reducing biliary colic pain than the hyoscine.

Other potential effects of CCK antagonists

A single animal study examined the effect of a CCK antagonist on the antinociceptive effect of the tricyclic antidepressant clomipramine in rats with streptozocin-induced diabetic neuropathy. Clomipramine on its own has the expected antinociceptive effect, as did the CCK antagonist. However, when both were given together the effect is compounded. Whether this effect is replicated in humans has not been examined, although with the well-known side effects associated with tricyclic use, the prospect of being able to enhance their analgesic effect while reducing the dose administered suggest that human studies are definitely needed.

Another prospective use of CCK antagonists is in the management of opioid withdrawal reactions. In rats treated on an ongoing basis with opioid in which naloxone is given to reverse the opioid effect, withdrawal reaction is precipitated. If these animals are treated with the CCK agonist caerulein, this reaction is increased while pretreatment with the CCK B antagonist L365,260 attenuates this withdrawal reaction. The human implications of this effect have not been examined.

Human use

Unfortunately there are no licensed CCK antagonists available in the US or UK. Previously proglumide was available in the UK and proved to be a particularly effective and safe medication. One is left with a considerable body of animal evidence that suggests utility for this group of compounds but with comparatively little human corroboration. That said, in my experience the success rate with proglumide treatment was such to suggest that it should be a first-line treatment option. It seemed to have the following potential uses:

1 It could be effective for neuropathic pain when taken alone (presumably by enhancing the analgesic effect of endogenous endorphins and enkephalins).

2 It could enhance the analgesic effect of codeine and tramadol in pain regardless of the etiology.

3 It could enhance the analgesic effect of morphine and prevent tolerance to its effect, regardless of the etiology of the pain.

4 It could reduce the pain of chronic pancreatitis in a proportion of patients with this condition.

Its role in the treatment of opioid withdrawal reactions and that in enhancing the analgesic effects of tricyclics also need further investigation so that the potential strengths of these effects can be put in context.

Perhaps the major reason why proglumide, for example, has not been more extensively investigated with a view to gaining a pain-related indication is because of the age of the compound itself (it was originally synthesized in the 1960s) and because pain-related patents were granted in the 1980s and have therefore long since expired. Consequently, no pharmaceutical firm will be prepared to invest the considerable amount of money in undertaking studies for the purpose of licence application if they cannot gain exclusivity of sales if an indication were granted because of the absence of an active patent.

Conclusions

The use of CCK antagonists are based on a strong stream of logic. The peptide CCK is released after neural injury and with chronic opioid use.

It has anti-opioid effects which can be blocked by treatment of a CCK antagonist. CCK antagonists enhance opioid-derived antinociception and curtail antinociceptive tolerance. However, largely because of patent-related issues CCK antagonists are not currently, and unfortunately may never be, available for human pain management.

My experience with the mixed CCK A and B antagonist proglumide in the treatment of many thousands of patients is that its use was associated with very few side effects and it enhanced the analgesia derived from tramadol, codeine, dihydrocodeine, and strong opioids with impressive regularity. Furthermore, it seemed to reduce analgesic tolerance associated with the use of these opioids. It is hoped that in the future more human work will be done to determine the place of CCK antagonists in human pain management. One further hopes that drugs such as proglumide will once again become available.

Bibliography

Bernstein ZP, Yucht S, Battista E et al. Proglumide as a morphine adjunct in cancer pain management. *J Pain Symptom Manage* 1998; 15: 314–20.

Bodnar RJ, Paul D, Pasternak GW. Proglumide selectively potentiates supraspinal mu opioid analgesia in mice. *Neuropharmacology* 1990; 29: 507–10.

Bras JM, Laporte A-M, Benoliel JJ et al. Effects of peripheral axotomy on cholecystokinin neurotransmission in the rat spinal cord. *J Neurochemistry* 1999; 72: 858–67.

Coudore-Civiale MA, Courteix C, Boucher M et al. Potentiation of morphine and clomipramine analgesia by cholecystokinin B antagonist CI988 in diabetic rats. *Neurosci Lett* 2000; 286: 37–40.

Coudore-Civiale M-A, Courteix C, Fialip J et al. Spinal effect of the cholecystokinin B receptor antagonist CI988 on hyperalgesia, allodynia and morphine induced analgesia in diabetic and mononeuropathic rats. *Pain* 2000; 88: 15–22.

Dourish CT, Hawley D, Iversen SD. Enhancement of morphine analgesia and prevention of morphine tolerance in the rat by the cholecystokinin antagonist L365,260. *Eur J Pharmacol* 1988; 147: 469–72.

Dourish CT, O'Neill MF, Coughlan J et al. The selective CCK B receptor antagonist L365,260 enhances morphine analgesia and prevents morphine tolerance in the rat. *Eur J Pharmacol* 1990; 176: 35–44.

Dourish CT, O'Neill MF, Schafer LW et al. The cholecystokinin receptor antagonist devazepide enhances morphine induced analgesia but not morphine induced respiratory depression in the squirrel monkey. *J Pharmacol Exp Ther* 1990; 255: 1158–65.

Faris PL, Komisaruk BR, Watkins LR, Mayer DJ. Evidence for the neuropeptide cholecystokinin as an antagonist of opiate analgesia. *Science* 1983; 219: 31–2.

Hoffmann O, Wiesenfeld-Hallin Z. The CCK B receptor antagonist CI988 reverses tolerance to morphine in rats. *Neuro Report* 1994; 5: 2565–8.

Idanpaan-Heikkila JJ, Guilbaud G, Kayser V. Prevention of tolerance to the antinociceptive effects of systemic morphine by a selective cholecystokinin B receptor antagonist in a rat model of peripheral neuropathy. *J Pharmacol Exp Ther* 1997; 282: 1366–72.

Innis RB, Snyder SH. Distinct cholecystokinin receptors in brain and pancreas. *Proc Natl Acad Sci USA* 1980; 77: 6917–21.

Ivy AC, Oldberg E. A hormonal mechanism for gall-bladder contraction and evacuation. *Am J Physiol* 1928; 86: 599–613.

Kissin I, Bright CA, Bradley EL. Acute tolerance to continuously infused alfentanil: the role of cholecystokinin and *N*-methyl-D-aspartate nitric oxide systems. *Anesth Analg* 2000; 91: 110–6.

Lavigne GJ, Hargreaves KM, Schmidt EA, Dionne RA. Proglumide potentiates morphine analgesia for acute postsurgical pain. *Clin Pharmacol Ther* 1989; 45: 666–73.

Lavigne GJ, Millington WR, Mueller GP. The CCK A and CCK B receptor antagonists, Devazepide and L365,260, enhance morphine antinociception only in non-acclimated rats exposed to a novel environment. *Neuropeptides* 1992; 21: 119–29.

Lehmann KA, Schlusener M, Arabatsis P. Failure of proglumide, a cholecystokinin antagonist, to potentiate clinical morphine analgesia. *Anesth Analg* 1989; 68: 51–6.

Linderfors N, Linden A, Brene Set al. CCK peptides and mRNA in the human brain. *Progress Neurobiology* 1993; 40: 671–90.

Lu L, Huang M, Liu Z, Ma L. Cholecystokinin B receptor antagonists attenuate morphine dependence and withdrawal in rats. *Neuro Report* 2000; 11: 829–32.

Lu L, Huang M, Ma L, Li J. Different role of cholecystokinin (CCK) A and CCK B receptors in relapse to morphine dependence in rats. *Behav Brain Res* 2001; 120: 105–10.

Malesci A, Pezzilli R, D'Amato M, Rovati L. CCK 1 receptor blockade for treatment of biliary colic: a pilot study. *Aliment Pharmacol Ther* 2003; 18: 333–7.

McCleane GJ. The cholecystokinin antagonist proglumide enhances the analgesic efficacy of morphine in humans with chronic benign pain. *Anesth Analg* 1998; 87: 1117–20.

McCleane GJ. The cholecystokinin antagonist proglumide has an analgesic effect in chronic pancreatitis. *Pancreas* 2000; 21: 324–5.

McCleane GJ. A phase 1 study of the cholecystokinin (CCK)B antagonist L365,260 in human subjects taking morphine for intractable non-cancer pain. *Neurosci Lett* 2002; 332; 210–12.

McCleane GJ. A randomised, double-blind, placebo controlled crossover study of the cholecystokinin 2 antagonist L365,260 as an adjunct to strong opioids in chronic human neuropathic pain. *Neurosci Lett* 2003; 338: 151–4.

McCleane GJ. The cholecystokinin antagonist proglumide enhances the analgesic effect of dihydrocodeine. *Clin J Pain* 2003; 19: 200–1.

McCleane GJ. Cholecystokinin antagonists in pain management. *Haworth Press.* Binghamton, USA, 2006.

Nichols ML, Bian D, Ossipov MH et al. Regulation of morphine anti allodynic efficacy by cholecystokinin in a rat model of neuropathic pain in rats. *J Pharmacol Exp Ther* 1995; 275: 1339–45.

Panerai AE, Rovati LC, Cocco E et al. Dissociation of tolerance and dependence to morphine: a possible role for cholecystokinin. *Brain Res* 1987; 410: 52–60.

Price DD, von der Gruen A, Miller J et al. Potentiation of systemic morphine analgesia in humans by proglumide, a cholecystokinin antagonist. *Anesth Analg* 1985; 64: 801–6.

Rady JJ, Holmes BB, Fujimoto JM. Antianalgesic action of dynorphin A mediated by spinal cholecystokinin. *Proc Soc Exp Biol Med* 1999; 220: 178–83.

Rady JJ, Lin W, Fujimoto JM. Pentobarbital antagonism of morphine analgesia mediated by spinal cholecystokinin. *J Pharmacol Exp Ther* 1998; 284: 878–85.

Rezvani A, Stokes KB, Rhoads DL, Way EL. Proglumide exhibits delta opioid agonist properties. *Alcohol Drug Res* 1987; 7: 135–46.

Schafer M, Zhou L, Stein C. Cholecystokinin inhibits peripheral opioid analgesia in inflamed tissue. *Neuroscience* 1998; 82: 603–11.

Schiffmann SN, Vanderhaeghen JJ. Distribution of cells containing mRNA encoding cholecystokinin in the rat central nervous system. *J Comparative Neurol* 1991; 304: 219–33.

Su HW, Kim Y-H, Choi YS, Song DK. Involvement of different subtypes of cholecystokinin receptors in opioid antinociception in the mouse. *Peptides* 1995; 16: 1229–34.

Tang J, Chou J, Iadarola M et al. Proglumide prevents and curtails acute tolerance to morphine in rats. *Neuropharmacology* 1984; 23: 715–8.

Tortorici V, Nogueira L, Salas R, Vanegas H. Involvement of local cholecystokinin in the tolerance induced by morphine microinjections into the periaqueductal gray of rats. *Pain* 2003; 102: 9–16.

Urban MO, Smith DJ, Gebhart GF. Involvement of spinal cholecystokinin B receptors in mediating Neurotensin hyperalgesia from the modularly nucleus raphe magnus in the rat. *J Pharmacol Exp Ther* 1996; 278: 90–8.

Valverde O, Maldonado R, Fournie-Zaluski MC, Roques BP. Cholecystokinin B antagonists strongly potentiate antinociception mediated by endogenous enkephalins. *J Pharmacol Exp Ther* 1994; 270: 77–88.

Watkins LR, Kinscheck IB, Mayer DJ. Potentiation of opiate analgesia and apparent reversal of morphine tolerance by proglumide. *Science* 1984; 224: 395–6.

Watkins LR, Kinscheck LB, Mayer DJ. Potentiation of morphine analgesia by the cholecystokinin antagonist proglumide. *Brain Res* 1985; 327: 169–80.

Wiesenfeld-Hallin Z, Xu X-J, Hughes J et al. PD134,308, a selective antagonist of cholecystokinin type B receptor, enhances the analgesic effect of morphine and synergistically interacts with intrathecal galanin to depress spinal nociceptive reflexes. *Proc Natl Acad Sci USA* 1990; 87: 7105–9.

Xu X-J, Alster P, Wu W-P et al. Increased level of cholecystokinin in cerebrospinal fluid is associated with chronic pain-like behaviour in spinally injured rats. *Peptides* 2001; 22: 1305–8.

Xu X-J, Puke MJ, Verge VM et al. Up regulation of cholecystokinin in primary sensory neurons is associated with morphine insensitivity in experimental neuropathic pain in the rat. *Neurosci Lett* 1993; 152: 129–32.

Yamamoto T, Sakashita Y. Differential effects of intrathecally administered morphine and its interaction with cholecystokinin B antagonists on thermal hyperalgesia following two models of experimental mononeuropathy in the rat. *Anesthesiology* 1999; 90: 1382–91.

Zarrindast M-R, Nikfar S, Rezayat M. Cholecystokinin receptor mechanism(s) and morphine tolerance in mice. *Pharmacology Toxicology* 1999; 84: 46–50.

Zarrindast M-R, Samiee F, Rezayat M. Antinociceptive effect of intracerebroventricular administration of cholecystokinin receptor agonist and antagonist in nerve ligated mice. *Pharmacol Ther* 2000; 87: 169–73.

Zarrindast M-R, Zabihi A, Rezayat M et al. Effects of caerulein and CCK antagonists on tolerance induced to morphine antinociception in mice. *Pharmacol Biochem Behav* 1997; 58: 173–8.

Zhang X, Dagerlind A, Elde E et al. Marked increase in cholecystokinin B receptor messenger RNA levels in rat dorsal root ganglia after peripheral axotomy. *Neuroscience* 1993; 57: 227–33.

Zhou X, Bayer BM. Increases of CCK mRNA and peptide in different brain areas following acute and chronic administration of morphine. *Brain Res* 1993; 625: 139–44.

Zhou Y, Sun Y-H, Zhang Z-W, Han J-S. Increased release of immunoreactive cholecystokinin octapeptide by morphine and potentiation of mu opioid analgesia by CCK B receptor antagonist L365,260 in rat spinal cord. *Eur J Pharmacol* 1993; 234: 147–54.

CHAPTER 13
Parenteral Anti-epileptics

Those involved in neurology and neurosurgical practice will be familiar with the use of intramuscular and intravenous (IV) anti-epileptic drugs (AEDs) for the treatment and prevention of epileptic seizures. Their use by those in purely pain practice is much less common.

Historically the first AED to be used in the treatment of pain was when phenytoin was used in the treatment of facial neuralgia in the early 1940s. Since that time oral phenytoin has been shown to be effective for the treatment of, among other conditions, painful diabetic neuropathy and so it is likely that it may be effective for other neuropathic pain conditions as well. Some concern must exist about the long-term use of oral phenytoin in view of its enzyme inducing, tachyphylactic, and gingival hyperplastic effects. With the advent of newer generation AEDs the long-term oral use of phenytoin must be questionable.

On the other hand, one is left with the problem of how to treat a patient with a flare-up of neuropathic pain, in whom a quick onset of treatment is desirable, or in whom the oral route is unavailable. What drugs can we use? Logically one would assume that if an oral formulation of a drug can be effective then the IV or intramuscular use of that same drug should have the same effect, and yet it was almost 60 years after the original description of the use of an AED in a patient with neuropathic pain before a study was published showing that IV infusion of phenytoin could also reduce neuropathic pain. Phenytoin was chosen as the parenteral AED as none of the newer AEDs were available in a parenteral formulation at that time. In this case the study compared the effect of a 2-h infusion of either phenytoin ($15\,mg\,Kg^{-1}$) or placebo in patients with neuropathic pain of mixed etiology. The interesting aspect of this study was not only that the IV phenytoin was effective, but also that after a 2-h infusion the duration of pain relief persisted for many days. Therefore the period of relief was longer than the duration of infusion and the half-life of the drug.

Pain Management: Expanding the Pharmacological Options, Gary J. McCleane. © 2008
Blackwell Publishing, ISBN: 978-1-4051-7823-5.

A further report of the successful use of IV phenytoin relates to its use in a patient with rapidly progressive neuropathic pain as a result of cancer.

However, while the parenteral formulation of phenytoin is a cheap and widely available drug, there are problems specific to the IV use of the drug. When diluted phenytoin is infused through a vein, should the cannula displace out of the vein then the spilt phenytoin can cause tissue ischemia and even skin necrosis. This can be of a severity to require surgical repair by debridement and skin-grafting. The reason for this toxicity is because of the very alkaline pH of the diluents accompanying phenytoin in the injectable form. These include potassium hydroxide and ethylene glycol.

With this in mind attention was focused on the manufacture of a safer version of phenytoin. This resulted in the marketing of fosphenytoin, a water soluble, ester pro-drug of phenytoin with near normal pH. When injected or infused, it requires activation by endogenous phosphatases before a therapeutic effect may be produced. While this increases markedly the safety of fosphenytoin, it does contribute to its major side effect. When injected, a burning sensation is produced in those areas of the body where phosphatases are found in the greatest concentration. In the male these are particularly prevalent in the groin and perineal areas and so an intense burning in that area often accompanies injection.

Perhaps the other very major drawback of fosphenytoin use is its expense. In the UK this amounts to about £40 (~$75) per ampoule.

Again, unsurprisingly, both the intramuscular and IV administration of fosphenytoin can produce pain relief in those with neuropathic pain. After intramuscular injection in patients with neuropathic pain of mixed etiology, pain relief of up to 48 h can be produced. When given by IV infusion over 24 h, again in patients with neuropathic pain of mixed etiology, pain relief is apparent with this relief extending to weeks. Indeed, a case report of a patient with neuropathic pain from operative intervention for a pelvic malignancy reports consistent pain relief of between 3 and 14 weeks after repeated 24-h infusions of fosphenytoin. The need for oral medication was significantly reduced during these periods of relief, and although infusion of phenytoin and fosphenytoin can both produce dizziness, nausea, and light-headedness, these persist for the infusion period and shortly after, whereas the side effects of oral medication, taken day-in, day-out, persist for the entire treatment period.

A further case report relates the successful alleviation of an acute flare-up of trigeminal neuralgia in three patients who had been refractory to other therapeutic interventions. In these three patients, relief persisted for several days after fosphenytoin use and allowed time for other oral pharmacotherapeutic strategies to be instituted. This exemplifies the potential benefit of parenteral AED in bringing about a rapid diminution of otherwise intractable pain.

Since fosphenytoin is a pro-drug of phenytoin, it would be expected that those who respond to phenytoin would respond to fosphenytoin and vice versa. In order not to confuse practitioners too much, a novel measurement unit is used for fosphenytoin. This is the "phenytoin equivalent unit" or PE unit, one of which is equal to 1 mg of phenytoin. The use of this was thought necessary since phenytoin and fosphenytoin are not milligram to milligram equal. Fosphenytoin is presented in vials of 500 PE in a volume of 10 ml. In the study examining intramuscular use, a dose of 500 PE was used, whereas in the IV study 1,500 PE diluted to 50 ml infused over 24 h was used.

It is likely that phenytoin and fosphenytoin achieve their analgesic effect by having sodium channel blocking actions. This they share with many other drugs used in pain practice such as carbamazepine, lidocaine, and mexiletine. It could therefore be argued that these other drugs could be used in place of phenytoin or fosphenytoin. However, clinical experience shows that phenytoin/fosphenytoin can be effective when these others drugs are ineffective: this may be because they target different sodium channels.

Possible clinical use

A number of clinical scenarios exist where parenteral fosphenytoin may be used:
- In a patient needing anti-epileptic drug treatment for neuropathic pain in whom the oral route is temporarily unavailable.
- In patients with neuropathic pain resistant to other available forms of therapy.
- In patients who derive sustained and protracted relief from a short-term infusion of fosphenytoin and in whom oral drug dose reduction accompanies relief from the fosphenytoin.
- As a "first aid" measure during an acute flare-up of neuropathic pain in an emergency room setting or by a General Practitioner in the patient's home (intramuscular, single dose use in place of, for example, strong opioid).

Conclusions

The parenteral formulations of phenytoin and fosphenytoin are among the few remedies for neuropathic pain which are available for intramuscular and IV use. When injected, the duration of relief may far outlive both the period of administration and the half-life of the drug. Phenytoin is familiar to many physicians and is cheap, but when given intravenously can produce skin necrosis if the drug spills outside the vein. In contrast, fosphenytoin is expensive, but lacks the risk of skin necrosis. From a purely results-based perspective, these drugs are interchangeable.

Bibliography

Chang VT. Intravenous phenytoin in the management of crescendo pelvic cancer-related pain. *J Pain Symptom Manage* 1997; 13: 238–40.

Cheshire WP. Fosphenytoin: an intravenous option for the management of acute trigeminal neuralgia crisis. *J Pain Symptom Manage* 2001; 21: 506–10.

McCleane GJ. Intramuscular fosphenytoin relieves neuropathic pain: a randomized, double-blind crossover study. *Analgesia* 1999; 4: 479–82.

McCleane GJ. Intravenous fosphenytoin relieves chronic neuropathic pain: a double-blind, placebo controlled crossover trial. *Analgesia* 2000; 5: 45–8.

McCleane GJ. Intravenous infusion of phenytoin relieves neuropathic pain: a randomized, double-blind, placebo-controlled, crossover study. *Anesth Analg* 2000; 90: 1007–8.

McCleane GJ. Intravenous infusion of fosphenytoin produces prolonged pain relief: a case report. *J Pain* 2002; 3: 156–8.

CHAPTER 14

Intravenous Lidocaine

The treatment of pain has improved immeasurably over the last few decades but there are still circumstances where our attempts to gain analgesia are thwarted by either therapeutic failure or production of intolerable side effects.

"Conventional" pharmacological treatment revolves around the use of acetaminophen, opioids and non-steroidal anti-inflammatories, with the use of antidepressants, anti-epileptics, membrane stabilizers and N-methyl-D-aspartate (NMDA) antagonists in particular circumstances, and requires the patients to either ingest or apply transdermally medication on a regular day-in, day-out basis. Where longer dosing intervals are appropriate, this is because extended release preparations are used. The aim is to achieve a steady state plasma concentration of the drug so that pain relief may be obtained. Unfortunately this may also expose the patient to day-in, day-out side effects with these side effects ranging from the trivial to the severe end of the spectrum and may be immediately obvious or more insidious.

The concept with the use of intravenous (IV) lidocaine is radically different. Here the drug is administered over a relatively short period of time and yet the potential relief lasts significantly beyond both the period of administration and the plasma half-life of this local anesthetic. Indeed, as will be described later, an infusion over a few hours can produce relief that extends to weeks and even months. Consequently, side effects, if any are apparent, are short-lived and last for a much shorter time than the pain relief. Indeed, IV lidocaine can be the sole analgesic, and between infusions the patient is essentially "drug free." A secondary potential benefit of IV lidocaine is that it may produce pain relief when all other modalities of pain treatment have failed.

It could therefore be argued that this concept has much appeal. However, it must be remembered that the use of IV lidocaine does not produce pain relief in all patients; but then again, neither does any other pain treatment.

Pain Management: Expanding the Pharmacological Options, Gary J. McCleane. © 2008
Blackwell Publishing, ISBN: 978-1-4051-7823-5.

In this chapter the following considerations will be examined:
- Mode of action of IV lidocaine
- The animal experimental evidence of an antinociceptive effect of systemic lidocaine
- The human experimental evidence of a pain relieving effect
- The human clinical evidence
- The safety (particularly cardiovascular safety) of IV lidocaine
- Suggested clinical use

Mode of action of local anesthetics

The intimate relationship between the activity of the membrane-bound enzyme $Na^+ - K^+$ ATPase and propagation of nerve impulses is firmly established. The ionic disequilibrium across semipermeable membrane in a nerve produces the potential energy for an action potential with the disequilibrium being rectified by the activity of $Na^+ - K^+$ ATPase. Local anesthetics block impulses by inhibiting individual Na^+ channels and thereby reducing the aggregate inward sodium current. When used at sufficient concentration, local anesthetics can cause complete neural blockade with obvious consequences on motor and sensory function of the nerve involved.

However, when agents such as lidocaine are administered systemically at lower doses, no effect is apparent on the conduction of action potentials in normal Aβ, Aδ, or C-primary afferents. In contrast, systemic lidocaine significantly suppresses the C-fiber evoked polysynaptic reflex generated by nerve stimulation. At concentrations of $1–20\,\mu g\ ml^{-1}$ lidocaine reversibly suppresses the tonic action potential discharge of acutely injured nerves and axotomized dorsal root ganglion cells.

Even when given in doses sufficient to cause significant cardiovascular side effects, lidocaine reduces the conduction in uninjured Aδ fibers by less than 5% and in C fibers by less than 50% demonstrating that when lidocaine is administered systemically at reasonable dose levels, "normal" neural function is uninterrupted, while a measurable effect is observed in damaged neural tissue.

It has also recently been shown that when lidocaine is administered systemically in animal models, sympathetic noradrenergic sprouting from damaged dorsal root ganglia is significantly reduced when compared to control animals. Of particular note is that this effect persists for more than 7 days after the cessation of lidocaine administration. This persistence of the effect from systemic lidocaine is again seen when frog sciatic nerves are treated with this drug causing a rapid, concentration-dependent decrease in the action potential plateau with this effect lasting for over 1 h after wash-out of lidocaine.

Therefore, in terms of the mechanistic effects of systemic lidocaine, it seems that this drug has a predominant effect on damaged neural tissue at concentrations well below those required to cause complete neural blockade, and that the effects of systemic lidocaine on neural activity can continue well beyond the period of drug administration.

Animal pain models

The use of spinal nerve root ligation in rats is a conventional method for producing allodynia, a cardinal feature of neuropathic pain, and allows the efficacy of pharmacological entities to be assessed as potential antineuro-pathic pain agents. When lidocaine is systemically infused for a defined period of time in rats with surgically induced allodynia, paw-withdrawal thresholds, a measure of allodynia, are increased for the period of infu-sion when low doses of lidocaine are administered. When larger doses are given, the reduction in allodynia persists well beyond the period of infusion. It has been noted that in some animals a dramatic reduc-tion in allodynia is observed while in others absolutely no effect is generated at all. This parallels human clinical practice closely. An alter-native model involves the creation of neuromas in rat sciatic nerves. Electrophysiological measurements can then be made to quantify the amount of spontaneous electrical activity that emanates from the neu-roma. Systemic lidocaine almost completely abolishes the spontaneous activity of these neuromas in the absence of nerve conduction blockade.

When given at the right concentrations, systemic lidocaine given to rats prior to the ligation of a sciatic nerve prevents the onset of thermal hyper-algesia. If the lidocaine is given 24 h after the ligation, then the thermal hyperalgesia already present is significantly reduced. Again thinking of rats with induced allodynia, systemic lidocaine causes up to a 66% reduc-tion in tactile allodynia. Remarkably, 21 days after the infusion period, 30–40% of the maximal possible effect on tactile allodynia persists.

The effect of IV lidocaine on allodynia (at least in animal models) seems to fall into three distinct phases. The first is a marked anti-allo-dynic effect during infusion that decreases in the 30–60 min after the ces-sation of infusion. The second is a transient reduction that occurs in the hours after infusion and the third is a sustained reduction developing in the 24 h after infusion that is maintained over the next 21 days.

It may be that IV lidocaine has effects other than the features of neu-ropathic pain. When used in animals undergoing colorectal distension, the electrophysiological responses suggest that there is a dose-dependent inhibition of visceromotor and cardiovascular reflexes evoked by colorectal distension suggesting a potentially beneficial effect on visceral pain.

It would seem fair to suggest that the animal evidence is in support of the contention that IV lidocaine can have a pain-relieving effect with the evidence being most robust in the case of neuropathic pain, but with a suggestion that a similar effect may be apparent in the case of visceral pain. Of particular note is that the effect of infusion in animal models can definitely far exceed the duration of infusion and the half-life of the drug, suggesting that the human clinical observation of prolonged relief has a scientific foundation and is not just a form of placebo response.

Human experimental pain

A small number of studies have examined the effect of IV lidocaine on human experimental pain. Two such experimental paradigms are the subcutaneous injection of capsaicin which causes an acute sensitization of the skin and the application of a heat stimulus. When these stimuli are applied and IV lidocaine administered, the area of secondary hyperalgesia as detected by brush strokes (but not that detected by filament application) is reduced. In an attempt to define whether the effect of the lidocaine is primarily peripheral or central, the effect of systemic IV and regional IV (by isolating the reference limb with a cuff) have been examined. After capsaicin application, both systemic and regional lidocaine slightly reduce capsaicin-related pain. The area of pin-prick hyperalgesia is significantly reduced after systemic but not after regional lidocaine treatment, suggesting that the effect of IV lidocaine is mediated centrally and not peripherally.

One other experimental model that has been utilized has been that of experimental skin burn in healthy volunteers. When such an injury is inflicted and lidocaine administered, by 12 h after infliction of the burn those treated with lidocaine had a significantly faster resolution of residual erythema compared to controls suggesting that it may have an effect on the long-term inflammation-induced tissues responses to thermal trauma.

Human clinical pain

Three recent systematic reviews have considered the available evidence of an analgesic effect when lidocaine is administered intravenously.

Challapalli and colleagues (2005) concluded:

> Lidocaine and oral analogs were safe drugs in controlled clinical trials for neuropathic pain, were better than placebo, and were as effective as other analgesics.

Tremont-Lukats and colleagues (2005) concluded:

> Lidocaine and mexiletine produced no major adverse events in controlled clinical trials, were superior to placebo to relieve neuropathic pain, and were as effective as other analgesics used for this condition.

Kalso and colleagues (1998) concluded in relationship to IV lidocaine that:

> Local anaesthetic-type drugs are effective in pain due to nerve damage…

Despite these conclusions the use of IV local anesthetics is not a mainstream practice. This is so because the concept is new. As long ago as 1943, Gordon reported the successful use of IV novocaine for the pain management of patients with burns. Since that time numerous reports have described the use of IV lidocaine in a broad spectrum of pain conditions. Unfortunately, as we will see, while these reports testify to an analgesic effect, few of the studies measure the absolute duration of effect of the IV treatment.

Neuropathic pain

In no other type of pain has IV lidocaine been more extensively studied than in neuropathic pain. Reports of its effects have been published in a range of conditions where this type of pain is manifest. Perhaps one of the most extensively studied of such conditions is painful diabetic neuropathy. When infused over several hours a definite pain-relieving effect is produced. In the study by Viola and colleagues (2006) 4-h infusions were given and pain parameters measured in the month subsequent to the next infusion. After these 4-h infusions, reductions in pain scores were recorded that persisted at day 14 and indeed day 28 after infusion.

Kastrup and colleagues (1987) also report that lidocaine infusions produced pain relief in their patients with painful diabetic neuropathy between 3 and 21 days after infusion.

Another commonly studied condition in which neuropathic pain is prominent is postherpetic neuralgia. Lidocaine appears to reduce both the pain and allodynia which characterize this condition. It has also been shown to reduce neuropathic pain of central origin, peripheral nerve injury, sciatica, and complex regional pain syndrome (type I). Both positive and negative results have been obtained when this treatment has been used in patients with spinal cord injury pain. Cahana and colleagues (2004) report their findings on positron emission tomography of a patient with central neuropathic pain who responded to IV lidocaine and in whom there was hypoactivity of the left posterolateral thalamus before treatment, which disappeared with therapy.

Postoperative pain

Historically, among the first reports of pain relief with IV local anesthetics was in the postoperative situation. As long ago as 1951, Keats and colleagues reported marked relief of postoperative pain when IV procaine was administered while in 1961 Bartlett and Hutaserani reported that of those 302 patients who received IV lidocaine during surgery, 83% experienced either no or little pain in the first 3 days after surgery as opposed to 25% of the 302 controls. More recently several studies have shown that when lidocaine is given intravenously during major abdominal surgery, postoperative morphine consumption is significantly reduced, as is movement pain and time to first bowel motion. The effects of the intraoperative lidocaine persist for the first 3 days after treatment. In addition, the release of cytokines during the trauma of surgery is also reduced by intraoperative lidocaine use.

Fibromyalgia

Several reports suggest that IV lidocaine can reduce the pain associated with fibromyalgia, a condition remarkable for its resistance to other forms of analgesic medication. These reports are of particular note, not only because they testify to an analgesic effect with IV lidocaine but also because of the duration of pain relief produced by infusion. In one study, daily lidocaine infusion produced pain relief that persisted until day 30 after treatment commenced, while in the other, over 40% of patients achieved between 13 and 18 weeks of pain relief after treatment.

Palliative care

A limited number of reports describe the use of IV lidocaine in terminally ill patients. Massey and colleagues (2002) report its use in a 5-year-old girl with metastatic retinoblastoma, the pain form which was resistant to opiates. IV lidocaine provided excellent pain relief without associated lethargy. Thomas and colleagues (2004) describe 82 patients of whom 82% reported a major response of their pain to lidocaine.

Postamputation pain

In a crossover trial of 32 patients with postamputation pain, Wu and colleagues (2002) compared the effect of IV lidocaine with morphine and placebo. Intravenous lidocaine reduced stump, but not phantom pain in this study.

Burns pain

As previously mentioned, IV procaine was initially attributed with an analgesic effect in burns patients. This pain-relieving effect is also possessed by lidocaine. When used in the acute phase after the initial burn, significant reductions in pain scores can be observed, and even the pain associated with wound-dressing changes can be reduced.

Other pain conditions

A number of reports suggest an analgesic effect when IV lidocaine is used in patients with chronic daily headache and proctalgia fugax.

Oral "local anesthetics"

One line of thought is that if a test dose of IV lidocaine produces a reduction in pain, then that effect can be replicated by oral mexiletine. Therefore a therapeutic trial with lidocaine gives a rapid answer to the question of the potential efficacy of mexiletine. While that may be a valid argument, it misses one of the salient points about the use of IV lidocaine, that the short-term administration of the drug can give prolonged relief and avoid the need, or at least minimize the need, to utilize other transdermal or oral medications on a day-in, day-out basis with the very real possibilities of the use of such medication producing ongoing side effects which compromise the quality of life of the patient. Mexiletine could not be considered a risk-free drug in terms of its propensity to cause adverse effects particularly as it is known to have a narrow therapeutic window.

It can be seen, therefore, that the use of IV lidocaine has been found to offer hope of pain reduction in a broad range of conditions giving rise to pain. Indeed, this is one of the major advantages of its use. Its effect is not dependent on the cause of the pain as it can reduce neuropathic pain, which arises from surgical trauma, burns muscles and so on.

Adverse effects

It would be naive not to think that many, if not most, practitioners will have significant anxiety about the use of parenteral lidocaine. From an early stage of training we are advised about toxic doses of local anesthetics which are significantly lower than what is suggested here. Undoubtedly local anesthetics can cause systemic side effects when used at excessive levels. More remarkable is the lack of significant side effects observed, for example, in over 8,000 IV infusions used in our pain practice. Indeed, while some patients do experience light-headedness and nausea, the most common side effect is phlebitis at the site of infusion. This is not related to the pH of the lidocaine or the presence or absence of preservatives and can be avoided if a glyceryl trinitrate patch (this anti-anginal has anti-inflammatory and analgesic effects) is placed above the infusion site.

Clearly, the major anxiety with IV lidocaine use is the worry about cardiovascular events. At least some of this anxiety may be generated by the association of its use in cardiology practice in the past where it was used as a cardiac anti-arrhythmic in postmyocardial infarction patients, among others. It should again be emphasized that in our own practice major cardiovascular side effects have not been observed, but clearly definitive clinical evidence of the cardiovascular safety of lidocaine is needed. In the past, if one wanted to measure cardiac output as a test of the positive or negative inotropic effect of a drug, major invasive testing was needed. It is now possible to measure cardiac outputs in a much less invasive fashion and one awaits studies of cardiac output measurement with IV lidocaine in non-cardiac pain patients.

Animal evidence of cardiac effect of IV lidocaine

Several studies on animals suggest that IV lidocaine has a negative inotropic effect mediated by an effect on sodium channels and calcium handling. However, in a human study of non-cardiac patients given up to $2\,mg\,kg^{-1}$ lidocaine intravenously, Matos and colleagues (1976) have shown that lidocaine had no effect on the strength of myocardial contractility. When it was given to dogs with induced coronary artery occlusion, the myocardial acidosis that normally occurs was reduced, and this may be mediated by a coronary artery dilating effect of lidocaine. As well as these effects, lidocaine increases the ventricular fibrillation threshold by a direct effect on ventricular cells.

This leaves a somewhat unsatisfactory situation. Extensive clinical experience suggests that IV lidocaine is a safe form of treatment and yet hard scientific evidence of such safety is missing. Conversely, hard scientific evidence of lack of safety is also absent. Perhaps, if work could be done to define the cardiovascular effects of IV lidocaine in non-cardiac patients at the doses used in pain management, then anxieties about the use of this treatment could be reduced.

Suggested clinical use

Unanswered questions about the clinical use of IV lidocaine

- Optimal dose
- Optimal infusion period
- Advantage of repeated infusions

From a clinical perspective, it seems that the quality and duration of response apparent after IV lidocaine use is more related to speed of infusion rather than absolute dose administered. The optimal dose and duration of infusion are not defined. In our practice we infuse either 1,200 mg lidocaine over 30 h or 1,000 mg over 7–9 h.

When a dose of 1,000 mg of lidocaine is given over 7–9 h it is provided as a 0.2% solution in dextrose (500 ml bags of this solution are commercially available) and the infusion takes place in a day-stay hospital setting.

When 1,200 mg is given over 30 h we utilize a disposable elastomeric infusion device with a pre-fixed infusion rate of $2 \, \text{ml h}^{-1}$ which is filled with 60 ml 2% lidocaine. A segment of a glyceryl trinitrate patch is placed about the infusion site to prevent thrombophlebitis and the infusor can then be placed in a pocket or up the sleeve of a shirt or blouse. Gravity is not needed for the infusion to run as the elastomeric device drives the infusate from the infusor into the vein. These infusions are given to patients who return home with them – hospital stay is not required.

Potential benefits of IV lidocaine

- Analgesia does not depend on source of pain
- Short-term administration can produce long-term pain relief
- Cheap
- Side effects can occur during infusion but do not persist despite long-term analgesic effect
- Can allow reduction or discontinuation of other analgesics with consequent reduction in drug-related side effects
- Treatment can be repeated, as required
- Can be provided on a domiciliary basis
- Analgesic tolerance appears not to occur with repeated infusions
- Ease of administration

Drawbacks to the use of IV lidocaine

- Not universally effective
- While extensive use suggests it is safe, hard evidence of safety (and particularly cardiovascular safety) not yet available
- Can cause infusion-related thrombophlebitis

Conclusions

It is accepted that many physicians will feel some unease about the IV administration of lidocaine. However, given the basic science evidence that underpins the contention that systemic lidocaine has an analgesic effect, it must merit consideration. Substantial clinical experience and a range of case reports and studies strongly suggest that IV lidocaine can have a pain-reducing effect in a broad range of conditions and that sustained pain relief can result from short-term infusion. During periods of pain relief after IV lidocaine administration, concomitant analgesics can be reduced or stopped with the consequent reduction in analgesic-related side effects. From a practical perspective, IV lidocaine can be administered by an IV infusion of variable durations, with the clinical impression that the quicker the speed of infusion the better the quality and more sustained the pain relief that may be produced. It could be argued that IV lidocaine is a possible therapy for any chronic pain condition with an efficacy rate at least that of any other analgesic option.

Bibliography

Abdi A, Lee DH, Chung JM. The anti-allodynic effects of amitriptyline, gabapentin, and lidocaine in a rat model of neuropathic pain. *Anesth Analg* 1998; 87: 1360–6.

Ackerman WE, Colclough GW, Juneja MM, Bellinger K. The management of oral mexiletine and IV lidocaine to treat chronic painful symmetrical distal diabetic neuropathy. *J Ky Med Assoc* 1991; 89: 500–1.

Araujo MC, Sinnott CJ, Strichartz GR. Multiple phases of relief from experimental mechanical allodynia by systemic lidocaine: responses to early and late infusions. *Pain* 2003; 103: 21–9.

Attal N, Gaudé V, Brasseur L et al. Intravenous lidocaine in central pain. A double-blind, placebo-controlled, psychophysical study. *Neurology* 2000; 54: 564–74.

Attal N, Rouaud J, Brasseur L et al. Systemic lidocaine in pain due to peripheral nerve injury and predictors of response. *Neurology* 2004; 62: 218–25.

Baranowski AP, De Courcey J, Bonello E. A trial of IV lidocaine on the pain and allodynia of postherpetic neuralgia. *J Pain Symptom Manage* 1999; 17: 429–33.

Bartlett EE, Hutaserani O. Xylocaine for the relief of postoperative pain. *Anesth Analg* 1961; 40: 296–304.

Bennett MI, Tai YM. Intravenous lignocaine in the management of primary fibromyalgia syndrome. *Int J Clin Pharmacol Res* 1995; 15: 115–19.

Burney RG, Di Fazio CA, Peach MJ et al. Anti-arrhythmic effects of lidocaine metabolites. *Am Heart J* 1974; 88: 765–9.

Butterworth JF, Strichartz GR. Molecular mechanisms of local anesthesia: a review. *Anesthesiology* 1990; 72: 711–34.

Cahana A, Carota A, Montadon ML, Annoni JM. The long-term effect of repeated IV lidocaine on central pain and possible correlation in positron emission tomography measurements. *Anesth Analg* 2004; 98: 1581–4.

Catterall WA. Common modes of drug action on Na$^+$ channels: local anesthetics, antiarrhythmics and anticonvulsants. *Trends Pharmacol Sci* 1987; 8: 57–65.

Chabal C, Russell LC, Burchiel KJ. The effect of IV lidocaine, tocainide, and mexiletine on spontaneously active fibers originating in rat sciatic neuromas. *Pain* 1989; 38: 333–8.

Challapalli V, Tremont-Lukats I, McNichol E et al. Systemic administration of local anesthetic agents to relieve neuropathic pain. *Cochrane Database Syst Rev* 2005; 4: CD003345.

Chaplan SR, Bach FW, Shafer SL, Yaksh TL. Prolonged alleviation of tactile allodynia by IV lidocaine in neuropathic rats. *Anesthesiology* 1995; 83: 775–85.

Devor M, Wall PD, Catalan N. Systemic lidocaine silences ectopic neuroma and DRG discharge without blocking nerve conduction. *Pain* 1992; 48: 261–8.

Dirks J, Fabricius P, Petersen KL et al. The effect of systemic lidocaine on pain and secondary hyperalgesia associated with the heat/capsaicin sensitization model in healthy volunteers. *Anesth Analg* 2000; 91: 967–72.

Finnerup NB, Biering-Sorensen F, Johannesen IL et al. Intravenous lidocaine relieves spinal cord injury pain: a randomized controlled trial. *Anesthesiology* 2005; 102: 1023–30.

Fujita Y, Endoh S, Yasukawa T, Sari A. Lidocaine increases the ventricular fibrillation threshold during bupivicaine-induced cardiotoxicity in pigs. *Br J Anaesth* 1998; 80: 218–22.

Furukawa T, Koumi S, Sakakibara Y et al. An analysis of lidocaine block of sodium current in isolated human atrial and ventricular myocytes. *J Mol Cell Cardiol* 1995; 27: 831–46.

Galer BS, Harle J, Rowbotham MC. Response to IV lidocaine infusion predicts subsequent response to oral mexiletine: a prospective study. *J Pain Symptom Manage* 1996; 12: 161–7.

Galer BS, Miller KV, Rowbotham MC. Response to IV lidocaine infusion differs based on clinical diagnosis and site of nervous system injury. *Neurology* 1993; 43: 1233–5.

Gee D, Wilson R, Angello D. Acute effect of lidocaine on coronary blood flow and myocardial function. *Angiology* 1990; 41: 30–5.

Gordon RA. Intravenous novocaine for analgesia in burns. *CMAJ* 1943; 49: 478–9.

Groudine SB, Fisher HA, Kaufman RP et al. Intravenous lidocaine speeds the return of bowel function, decreases postoperative pain, and shortens hospital stay in patients undergoing radical retropubic prostatectomy. *Anesth Analg* 1998; 86: 235–9.

Hand PJ, Stark RJ. Intravenous lignocaine infusions for severe chronic daily headache. *Med J Aust* 2000; 172: 157–9.

Hille B. Common mode of action of three agents that decrease the transient change in sodium permeability in nerves. *Nature* 1966; 210: 1220–2.

de Jong RH, Nace RA. Nerve impulse conduction during IV lidocaine injection. *Anesthesiology* 1968; 29: 22–8.

Jönsson A, Cassuto J, Hanson B. Inhibition of burn pain by IV lignocaine infusion. *Lancet* 1991; 338: 151–2.

Kalso E, Tramer MR, McQuay HJ, Moore RA. Systemic local-anaesthetic-type drugs in chronic pain: a systematic review. *Eur J Pain* 1998; 2: 3–14.

Kastrup J, Petersen P, Dejgård A et al. Intravenous lidocaine infusion – a new treatment of chronic painful diabetic neuropathy. *Pain* 1987; 28: 69–75.

Kastrup J, Bach FW, Petersen P et al. Lidocaine treatment of painful diabetic neuropathy and endogenous opioid peptides in plasma. *Clin J Pain* 1989; 5: 239–44.

Keats AS, D'Alessandro G, Beecher HK. A controlled study of pain relief by IV procaine. *JAMA* 1951; 147: 1761–3.

Khodorova A, Meissner K, Leeson S, Strichartz GR. Lidocaine selectively blocks abnormal impulses arising from noninactivating Na channels. *Muscle Nerve* 2001; 24: 634–47.

Koppert W, Ostermeier N, Sittl R et al. Low-dose lidocaine reduces secondary hyperalgesia by a central mode of action. *Pain* 2000; 85: 217–24.

Koppert W, Weigand M, Neumann F et al. Perioperative IV lidocaine has preventative effects on postoperative pain and morphine consumption after major abdominal surgery. *Anesth Analg* 2004; 98: 1050–5.

Kuo CP, Jao KM, Wong CS et al. Comparison of the effects of thoracic epidural analgesia and i.v. infusion with lidocaine on cytokine response, postoperative pain and bowel function in patients undergoing colonic surgery. *Br J Anaesth* 2006; 97: 640–6.

Kvarnstrom A, Karisten R, Quiding H, Gordh T. The analgesic effect of IV ketamine and lidocaine on pain after spinal cord injury. *Acta Anaesthesiol Scand* 2004; 48: 498–506.

Massey GV, Pedigo S, Dunn NL et al. Continuous lidocaine infusion for the relief of refractory malignant pain in a terminally ill pediatric cancer patient. *J Pediatr Hematol Oncol* 2002; 24: 566–8.

Matos L, Hankoczy J, Torok E. Effects of lidocaine on myocardial function and on isoprenaline induced circulatory changes in man. *Int J Clin Pharmacol Biopharm* 1976; 14: 83–91.

Matsumura N, Matsumura H, Abiko Y. Effect of lidocaine on the myocardial acidosis induced by coronary artery occlusion in dogs. *J Pharmacol Exp Ther* 1987; 1114–19.

Mattsson U, Cassuto J, Tarnow P et al. Intravenous lidocaine infusion in the treatment of experimental human skin burns – digital color image analysis of erythema development. *Burns* 2000; 26: 710–15.

Medrik-Goldberg T, Lifschitz D, Pud D et al. Intravenous lidocaine, amantadine, and placebo in the treatment of sciatica: a double-blind, randomized, controlled study. *Reg Anesth Pain Med* 1999; 24: 534–40.

Ness TJ. Intravenous lidocaine inhibits visceral nociceptive reflexes and spinal neurons in the rat. *Anesthesiology* 2000; 92: 1685–91.

Pankucsi C, Varró A, Nánási PP. Three distinct components of the negative inotropic action of lidocaine in dog Purkinje fiber. *Gen Pharmacol* 1996; 27: 69–71.

Peleg R, Shvartzman P. Low-dose IV lidocaine as treatment for proctalgia fugax. *Reg Anesth Pain Med* 2002; 27: 97–9.

Raphael JH, Southall JL, Treharne GJ, Kitas GD. Efficacy and adverse effects of IV lignocaine therapy in fibromyalgia syndrome. *BMC Musculoskeletal Disorders* 2002; 3: 1–8.

Rowbotham MC, Reisner-Keller LA, Fields HL. Both IV lidocaine and morphine reduce the pain of postherpetic neuralgia. *Neurology* 1991; 41: 1024–8.

Sinnott CJ, Garfield JM, Strichartz GR. Differential efficacy of IV lidocaine in alleviating ipsilateral versus contralateral neuropathic pain in the rat. *Pain* 1999; 80: 521–31.

Smith LJ, Shih A, Miletic G, Miletic V. Continual systemic infusion of lidocaine provides analgesia in an animal model of neuropathic pain. *Pain* 2002; 97: 267–73.

Tanelian DL, MacIver MB. Analgesic concentrations of lidocaine suppress tonic A-delta and C fiber discharges produced by acute injury. *Anesthesiology* 1991; 74: 934–6.

Taylor RE. Effect of procaine on electrical properties of squid axon membrane. *Am J Physiol* 1959: 196; 1071–8.

Thomas J, Kronenberg R, Cox MC et al. Intravenous lidocaine relieves severe pain: results of an inpatient hospice chart review. *J Palliat Med* 2004; 7: 660–7.

Tremont-Lukats IW, Challapalli V, McNichol ED et al. Systemic administration of local anesthetics to relieve neuropathic pain: a systematic review and meta-analysis. *Anesth Analg* 2005; 101: 1738–49.

Tremont-Lukats IW, Hutson PR, Backonja MM. A randomized, double-masked, placebo-controlled pilot trial of extended IV lidocaine infusion for relief of ongoing neuropathic pain. *Clin J Pain* 2006; 22: 266–71.

Viola V, Newnham HH, Simpson RW. Treatment of intractable painful diabetic neuropathy with IV lidocaine. *J Diabetes Complications* 2006; 20: 34–9.

Wallace MS, Ridgeway BM, Leung AY et al. Concentration-effect relationship of IV lidocaine on the allodynia of complex regional pain syndrome type I and II. *Anesthesiology* 2000; 92: 75–83.

Williams DR, Stark RJ. Intravenous lignocaine (lidocaine) infusion for the treatment of chronic daily headache with substantial medication overuse. *Cephalgia* 2003; 23: 963–71.

Wilson RA, Soei LK, Bezstarosti K et al. Negative inotropy of lidocaine: possible biochemical mechanisms. *Eur Heart J* 1993; 14: 284–9.

Woolf CJ, Wiesenfeld-Hallin Z. The systemic administration of local anaesthetics produces a selective depression of C-afferent fibre evoked activity in the spinal cord. *Pain* 1985; 23: 361–74.

Wu CL, Tella P, Staats PS et al. Analgesic effects of IV lidocaine and morphine on postamputation pain: a randomized double-blind, active placebo-controlled, crossover trial. *Anesthesiology* 2002; 96: 841–8.

Zhang J-M, Li H, Munir MA. Decreasing sympathetic sprouting in pathologic sensory ganglia: a new mechanism for treating neuropathic pain using lidocaine. *Pain* 2004; 109: 143–9.

CHAPTER 15

L-Carnitine

L-Carnitine is a quaternary ammonium compound synthesized from the amino acids lysine and methionine primarily in the liver and kidneys. In vivo it has a role in transporting fatty acids from the cytosol to the mitochondria but an increasing body of evidence suggests that it may also have a useful effect on the neuropathic pain produced by a number of conditions. In the UK it is widely sold as a nutritional supplement to which a number of benefits are attributed, including weight loss, reduction in depression, and even an effect on the mental decline that accompanies aging. In other countries, such as Canada, products containing L-carnitine cannot be marketed as "natural health products", as it is not considered a natural ingredient.

Mechanism of effect of carnitine

A number of modes of action of carnitine in relationship to its antinociceptive effect have been proposed. One of these relates to the observation that in rats with induced diabetes the content of substance P, an important pain-related neurotransmitter, is reduced in the sciatic nerve and lumbar spinal cord and that this decrease found with the onset of diabetes can be prevented by carnitine pretreatment.

More recently it has been shown that carnitine has an effect on the expression of metabotropic glutamate receptors (mGlu) in lamina II, III, and IV of the spinal cord and cerebral cortex. The increase in immunoreactivity in these parts is for mGlu 1 and 2 receptors and not for the others in this family. Dorsal root ganglia cell culture techniques have now shown that the up-regulation of mGlu expression involves transcriptional activation mediated by nuclear factor-kappaB (NF-kappaB). Indeed in these cell culture models, a single application of carnitine causes a rapid and transient increase in mGlu2 representation.

Pain Management: Expanding the Pharmacological Options, Gary J. McCleane. © 2008 Blackwell Publishing, ISBN: 978-1-4051-7823-5.

Animal experimental evidence of antinociceptive effect of carnitine

A number of experimental techniques have shown that carnitine can have an antinociceptive effect. These studies have concentrated on examining the actions of carnitine in chemotherapy-induced and diabetic neuropathic pain as well as on an acute pain model.

An unfortunate consequence of the use of certain chemotherapeutic agents in cancer patients is their propensity to cause neuropathy and indeed neuropathic pain. A positive effect has been demonstrated when animals are treated with carnitine and these chemotherapeutic agents are administered. Among the chemotherapy agents known to cause neuropathic pain which can be lessened by carnitine are paclitaxel, oxaliplatin, cisplatin, and vincristine.

In one study, paclitaxel was administered intraperitoneally to rats which induced marked mechanical hypersensitivity. When carnitine was co-administered with the paclitaxel, pain was prevented and this preventative effect persisted for up to 3 weeks after the last administration of carnitine. In those rats treated initially only with paclitaxel and in whom mechanical hypersensitivity is induced, subsequent carnitine significantly reduced nociception. These results are confirmed in other studies and suggest that carnitine treatment can have both a preventative and antinociceptive effect when used in animals treated with certain chemotherapy agents. Crucially, given the context in which these cancer chemotherapy agents are used, carnitine treatment has no effect on the chemotherapy agents' antitumor properties.

Carnitine has also been studied in the diabetic field. When carnitine is given to rats with streptozotocin-induced diabetes, the autonomic neuropathy that normally accompanies the diabetes is prevented.

A single study has examined the effect of carnitine on acute pain using a mouse hot-plate test and a rat paw-pressure test. In both carnitine-treated mice and rats an increase in pain threshold was observed after 7 days of treatment. Furthermore, carnitine reversed the normal hyperalgesia found after NMDA administration. When the unselective muscarinic antagonist atropine is given to carnitine-treated animals, the normal increase in nociceptive threshold is prevented. However, that antinociceptive effect of carnitine is unaltered by opioid antagonist naloxone, a GABA B antagonist, and by a monoamine synthesis inhibitor, suggesting a crucial role of muscarinic receptors in the antinociceptive effect of carnitine.

Carnitine in human pain

An increasing number of human studies demonstrate that carnitine treatment reduces neuropathic pain and that its use is uncomplicated by severe adverse effects. Particular examination has been made into the effect of carnitine on the pain associated with human immunodeficiency virus (HIV). Infection with HIV can be complicated by a painful symmetrical neuropathy the pain of which can be lessened by parenteral and oral carnitine. More commonly the treatments for HIV can lead to a significant neuropathy and neuropathic pain. Nucleoside analog reverse transcriptase inhibitors (NRTIs) disrupt mitochondrial DNA synthesis impairing energy metabolism and are widely used in the management of patients with HIV. Their use is also complicated by an antiretroviral toxic neuropathy. Studies have shown that long-term carnitine treatment produces symptomatic improvement in most patients with neuropathic pain while allowing the continued use of the antiretroviral medication. Furthermore, significant adverse effects of carnitine treatment are rare. In one study skin biopsies were taken before and during long-term carnitine treatment with patients taking antiretroviral medication. It was noted that not only were the symptoms of the medication-related neuropathy improved but also peripheral nerve regeneration accompanied carnitine treatment.

The other clinical field in which carnitine has been tested is that of painful diabetic neuropathy. When carnitine is given over the long term, painful diabetic neuropathy is reduced while regeneration occurs in peripheral nerve tissue. Although nerve conduction velocities and amplitudes do not improve with treatment, vibration sense does.

We have utilized carnitine treatment in our own practice for a number of years for patients with neuropathic pain regardless of etiology and have found it to be useful in reducing pain without the complication of significant side effects in many patients. Usually it causes a noticeable, but not complete, reduction in pain with the degree of pain relief being somewhat less than, say, with AEDs, but occurring more frequently than when other drug classes are used. Because of its ease of tolerability a high proportion of patients elect to continue the use of the drug in contrast with many other therapeutic options.

When a suggestion of use is made to a patient we recommend they take L-carnitine 500 mg twice daily for a 2-week period. If no effect is apparent after this time, then it is discontinued.

Conclusions

Carnitine is unusual among the agents that can be effective in the treatment of neuropathic pain in that it is not a prescribable medication, but rather one which the patient has to purchase for themselves. Despite not being a mainstream treatment, there seems to be a strength of experimental evidence rationalizing how it may have an analgesic effect supported by animal experimental evidence of an antinociceptive effect along with human clinical evidence from certain well-defined neuropathic pain condition. What is lacking is evidence, other than that of an anecdotal nature, regarding its effect in other human neuropathic and non-neuropathic conditions although there is strong impression that it is of use in a wide spectrum of neuropathic and non-neuropathic conditions, including, for example, fibromyalgia. Patients seem keen on this alternative as it is marketed as a dietary supplement that can cause weight loss and reduce depression and since many other analgesic agents cause weight gain and long-term pain can precipitate depression, these additional potential benefits are of attraction. Its lack of sedative effects also appeals.

Bibliography

Chiechio S, Caricasole A, Barletta E et al. L-Acetylcarnitine induces analgesia by selectively up-regulating mGlu2 metabotropic glutamate receptors. *Mol Pharmacol* 2002; 61: 989–96.

Chiechio S, Copani A, De Petris L et al. Transcriptional regulation of metabotropic glutamate receptor 2/3 expression by the NF-kappaB pathway in primary dorsal root ganglia neurons: a possible mechanism for the analgesic effect of L-acetylcarnitine. *Mol Pain* 2006; 2: 20.

Di Giulio AM, Gorio A, Bertelli A et al. Acetyl-L-carnitine prevents substance P loss in the sciatic nerve and lumbar spinal cord of diabetic animals. *Int J Clin Pharmacol Res* 1992; 12: 243–6.

Flatters SJ, Xiao WH, Bennett GJ. Acetyl-L-carnitine prevents and reduces paclitaxel-induced painful peripheral neuropathy. *Neurosci Lett* 2006; 397: 219–23.

Ghelardini C, Galeotti N, Calvani M et al. Acetyl-L-carnitine induces muscarinic antinociception in mice and rats. *Neuropharmacology* 2002; 43: 1180–7.

Ghirardi O, Lo Giudice P, Pisano C et al. Acetyl-L-carnitine prevents and reverts experimental chronic neurotoxicity induced by oxaliplatin, without altering its antitumor properties. *Anticancer Res* 25: 2681–7.

Ghirardi O, Vertechy M, Vesci L et al. Chemotherapy-induced allodynia: neuroprotective effect of acetyl-L-carnitine. *In Vivo* 2005; 19: 631–7.

Hart AM, Wilson AD, Montovani C et al. Acetyl-L-carnitine: a pathogenesis based treatment for HIV-associated antiretroviral toxic neuropathy. *AIDS* 2004; 18: 1549–60.

Herzmann C, Johnson MA, Youle M. Long-term effect of acetyl-L-carnitine for antiretroviral toxic neuropathy. *HIV Clin Trials* 2005; 6: 344–50.

La Giudice P, Careddu A, Magni G et al. Autonomic neuropathy in streptozotocin diabetic rats: effect of acetyl-L-carnitine. *Diabetes Res Clin Pract* 2002; 56: 173–80.

Noofri M, Fulgente T, Melchionda D et al. L-Acetylcarnitine as a new therapeutic approach for peripheral neuropathies with pain. *Int J Clin Pharmacol Res* 1995; 15: 9–15.

Osio M, Muscia F, Zampini L et al. Acetyl-L-carnitine in the treatment of painful antiretroviral toxic neuropathy in human immunodeficiency virus patients: an open label study. *J Peripher Nerv Syst* 2006; 11: 72–6.

Pisano C, Pratesi G, Laccabue D et al. Paclitaxel and Cisplatin-induced neurotoxicity: a protective role of acetyl-L-carnitine. *Clin Cancer Res* 2003; 9: 5756–67.

Scarpini E, Sacilotto G, Baron P et al. Effect of acetyl-L-carnitine in the treatment of painful peripheral neuropathies in HIV+ patients. *J Peripher Nerv Syst* 1997; 2: 250–2.

Sima AA, Calvani M, Mehra M, Amato A. Acetyl-L-carnitine improves pain, nerve regeneration, and vibratory perception in patients with chronic diabetic neuropathy. *Diabetes Care* 2005; 28: 96–101.

Youle M, Osio M. A double-blind, parallel-group, placebo-controlled, multicenter study of acetyl-L-carnitine in the symptomatic treatment of antiretroviral toxic neuropathy in patients with HIV-1 infection. *HIV Med* 2007; 8: 241–50.

CHAPTER 16

Other Pharmacological Options (Botulinum, Cimetidine, Glucosamine)

Although complete chapters have been dedicated to a variety of individual and classes of medication, there are a number of other options for whom the supportive evidence is not quite as strong or whose use, despite being largely "off-label," is already mainstream. In this chapter some of these other pharmacological options will be discussed. It is not designed to be a comprehensive list of alternatives but rather a mechanism to highlight those options which have proven to be of value in clinical practice.

Adenosine

A variety of adenosine receptors exist both in the peripheral and central nervous systems. These subserve both anti- and pro-nociceptive effects. In animal models, administration of adenosine A_1 agonists, or of inhibitors of adenosine kinase (which increase tissue levels of adenosine), has an antinociceptive effect by interaction with these A_1 receptors. In addition, adenosine kinase inhibitors can also have an anti-inflammatory effect by interacting with A_{2A} receptors on peripheral immune cells. In theory, adenosine administration could have a pain-facilitating effect by actions on A_{2B} and A_3 receptors on mast cells, but in practice these receptors have a lower affinity for adenosine than the A_1 receptors. Another potential issue is that there may be species differences in the actions of the individual adenosine receptors.

In human experimental pain models, the intravenous (IV) administration of adenosine reduces central sensitization. Clinical studies suggest that the IV infusion of adenosine at a dose of $50\,\mu g\,kg^{-1}\,min^{-1}$ over 60 min can significantly reduce the area over which tactile allodynia is felt without reducing spontaneous pain. In one of these studies a single adenosine infusion reduced pain in three patients for 5, 16, and 25 months.

Pain Management: Expanding the Pharmacological Options, Gary J. McCleane. © 2008
Blackwell Publishing, ISBN: 978-1-4051-7823-5.

Perhaps one of the greatest drawbacks of IV adenosine use is the cost of the drug.

Baclofen

Baclofen has gained popularity in the treatment of muscle spasm and can be administered orally or by intrathecal infusion. It achieves muscle relaxation by virtue of its gamma amino butyric acid (GABA) agonist properties and is commendable as a muscle relaxant because of its speed of onset, effective antispasmodic action, and low incidence of side effects.

Baclofen could be considered as a first-line treatment for muscle spasm. But it has one other action as well and that is as a treatment of trigeminal neuralgia. When used for this condition it can be administered in two fashions. The first is as a long-term treatment where its benefit would be a superior tolerability to many AEDs and the second being in the management of a flare-up of this neuralgia. Many patients will be taking long-term treatment for trigeminal neuralgia in the hope that it may prevent, or at least reduce, the occurrence of flare-ups but are left with the dilemma of what to take if their trigeminal neuralgia becomes acutely worse. Baclofen, with which there is no need to titrate up a dose but rather commence a hopefully therapeutic dose from the start, can be used during flare-ups because of its quick onset time.

When used in practice, for most healthy adults a dose of 10 mg baclofen thrice daily can be used with a reduced dose being selected in the frail. If 10 mg thrice daily is insufficient, then it can be increased up to 20 mg thrice daily by the oral route.

Botulinum toxin

Botulinum toxin is a product of the anaerobe *Clostridium botulinum* and is indicated for the treatment of cervical dystonia, blepharospasm, hemifacial spasm, axillary hyperhidrosis, and glabellar wrinkles. A number of immunologically distinct serotypes exist of which type A and type B are the predominant forms in clinical practice. At least some of its effect is due to its ability to inhibit release of acetylcholine from cholinergic nerve terminals. In addition, it has been suggested that it may also inhibit glutamate release, as well as that of calcitonin gene-related peptide and substance P. Animal experimentation has shown that, as well as having muscle relaxant effects, botulinum toxin type A can have marked anti-allodynic effects after a single injection which persists for up to 3 weeks in a chronic nerve constriction model of neuropathic pain. In addition, it can reduce both the acute and chronic response to formalin injection in a rat paw.

As well as those conditions for which it has an indication, there are a number of others for which evidence, of varying strengths, exists for a pain-reducing effect:

- Migraine
- Cluster headache
- Chronic daily headache
- Piriformis muscle spasm
- Tension headache
- Temperomandibular joint dysfunction
- Chronic low back pain
- Lateral epicondylitis
- Myofascial pain
- Carpal tunnel syndrome
- Complex regional pain syndrome
- Postherpetic neuralgia
- Spinal cord injury pain
- Joint pain

It should be emphasized that some of the reports of successful use of botulinum toxin in these conditions report its use in a small number of patients and therefore its use in these conditions is speculative rather than heavily evidence based.

Perhaps one of the most unusual pain uses of botulinum toxin is that of intra-articular injection in patients with refractory joint pain with refractory being defined as unresponsive to conventional oral and intra-articular therapy. In one report of just eleven patients, five with osteoarthritis, five with rheumatoid arthritis, and one with psoriatic arthritis, maximal relief was seen with shoulder injection, while lower extremity joint injection was associated with a lesser, but clinically useful, reduction in pain and increase in range of movements. The duration of pain relief ranged from 3 to 12 months.

It would seem that given the well-proven effects of botulinum toxin on specific types of muscle spasm that it should be considered in conditions where any muscle spasm is present. The benefits of use include one-off injections that may give prolonged relief and the possibility of reducing or stopping orally administered muscle relaxant medication.

Cimetidine

Cimetidine is well known for its anti-ulcer effect produced by its ability to block H_2 receptors. It can also decrease calcium levels and produce a reduction in symptoms of patients with hyperparathyroidism. Chronic calcific tendonitis of the shoulder is a disabling and painful condition which responds relatively poorly to analgesic intervention. In a study of 16 patients with this condition, Yokoyama and colleagues (2003) found that cimetidine at a dose of 200 mg twice daily for a 3-month period in patients resistant to conservative treatment caused a significant and marked decrease in pain with 63% of patients becoming pain free. Radiological evidence of calcification of the tendon disappeared in 56% and decreased in a further 25% of treated patients. Therefore, in this small study, only 19% of patients failed to achieve at least a partial reduction in the calcification of the tendon. These patients were reviewed after 4 and 24 months and all were found to be still improved. The mechanism of this beneficial effect of cimetidine is unclear.

Clonazepam

Clonazepam is recognized as a treatment for epilepsy and in particular status epilepticus where it is given as an IV infusion. In addition to its anticonvulsant properties, clonazepam has several other potentially useful properties. Clonazepam can reduce muscle spasm, induce sleep, and reduce neuropathic pain with an impression that it is most effective for lancinating pain. In addition, it has amnesic and anti-anxiety effects. One would expect that with its long half-life that if taken on a regular basis, even if only at night, the day-time sedation would complicate its use. In practice, while such sedation may occur, it is not universal.

Clonazepam, 05–1.5 mg, at night can be useful as an aid to sleep, particularly in patients where muscle spasm or lancinating pain is problematical and where the patient is of an anxious disposition. Its hypnotic effects make it an alternative to a tricyclic antidepressant which is often used to improve sleep.

Case reports also suggest that clonazepam can be useful in the management of phantom limb pain and myofascial pain syndrome, and when used topically as an oral rinse in the treatment of stomatodynia.

Glucosamine

Glucosamine is a precursor in proteoglycan synthesis. This preparation is widely available for purchase by the public and has gained popularity for its effect on joint pain. Its use was widespread before scientific investigation gave support for its reputed effects. It is now thought that glucosamine may achieve a number of goals. First, it may reduce pain and stiffness in an affected joint. Second, it may prevent progression of the osteoarthritic process in a joint as evidenced by an increase, rather than decrease, in articular cartilage thickness, and third, it may have a protective effect on other unaffected joints.

The majority of clinical studies have examined its use in the treatment of osteoarthritis of the knee and the consensus is that glucosamine has a moderate effect of pain and stiffness. The question remains, however, if glucosamine does have a positive effect on knee osteoarthritis, could it also have an effect on osteoarthritis in other joints? In terms of hard scientific evidence this question must remain open. However, from an anecdotal perspective there is no doubt that glucosamine can ease symptoms in any osteoarthritic joint. Indeed, why would it not have an effect on all joints and not just the knee?

In clinical practice a normal dose of glucosamine would be 1500 mg daily, taken either as a single, or in divided doses. It is presented in tablet and sachet forms and is prepared from bovine cartilage or shellfish. Some patients experience benefit within days of treatment commencement, whereas in others it may be many months before a gradual decrease in symptoms are observed. Therefore patients should be instructed that treatment needs to be long term. Many patients like the concept that glucosamine actually replaces worn away cartilage rather than just masking the pain from a damaged joint. In addition, its lack of significant side effects is also of appeal.

Unfortunately for the patient, when they go to purchase glucosamine, it is often presented with a bewildering variety of additives including omega-fish oils, chondroitin, and so on. While these may offer additional benefit, their effects are not yet fully established.

Hyaluronidase

This naturally occurring enzyme has long been used to help the disbursement of fluid in tissues. It is also used in local anesthetic techniques to help penetration of local anesthetic to nerve tissue.

Several case reports describe the use of intrathecal Hyaluronidase in the treatment of arachnoiditis where it is assumed that it helps the breakdown of fine adhesions. In my practice we also use it by the epidural route in patients with failed back surgery syndrome and epidural fibrosis where again it may help the breakdown of fine scar tissue but clearly not of more dense adhesions. In this use it quite often gives pain relief that extends to several months with a combination of 3,000 IU Hyaluronidase along with 35 ml 0.025% bupivicaine being used. Given the lack of serious adverse effects with its use, it can be repeated indefinitely, in contrast to the epidural use of corticosteroids. For convenience, we tend to use the caudal epidural route rather than a formal lumbar epidural which may be a more difficult procedure in a patient with previous back surgery.

One other use of Hyaluronidase is for tender point injection where its effect may be comparable to that obtained with corticosteroid injection, but again without the possible long-term consequences of corticosteroid use.

Side effects with Hyaluronidase use are extremely infrequent. On one occasion I have witnessed a mild allergic reaction with its use.

Conclusions

A variety of uses for drugs have been described here with many of these uses being at the anecdotal, rather than evidence-based end of the spectrum. That said, clinical use has suggested much merit with their use and a low risk of adverse effects. It is unlikely with many of them that they will ever obtain a specific indication for the pain uses described and yet it would be a great shame if the knowledge of their potential effectiveness fades from view.

Bibliography

Adenosine
Belfrage M, Solevi A, Segerdahl M et al. Systemic adenosine infusion alleviates spontaneous and stimulus evoked pain in patients with peripheral neuropathic pain. *Anesth Analg* 1995; 81: 713–17.

Chizh BA, Dusch M, Puthawala M et al. The effect of IV infusion of adenosine on electrically evoked hyperalgesia in a healthy volunteer model of central sensitization. *Anesth Analg* 2004; 99: 816–22.

Hayashida M, Fukuda K, Fukunaga A. Clinical application of adenosine and ATP for pain control. *J Anesth* 2005; 19: 225–35.

Lynch ME, Clark AJ, Sawynok J. IV adenosine alleviates neuropathic pain: a double blind placebo controlled crossover trial using an enriched enrolment design. *Pain* 2003; 103: 111–17.

Sjolund KF, Belfrage M, Karlsten R et al. Systemic adenosine infusion reduces the area of tactile allodynia in neuropathic pain following peripheral nerve injury: a multicentre, placebo-controlled study. *Eur J Pain* 2001; 5: 199–207.

Baclofen
Fromm GH, Terrence CF, Chattha AS. Baclofen in the treatment of trigeminal neuralgia: double-blind study and long-term follow-up. *Ann Neurol* 1984; 15: 240–4.

Parmar BS, Shah KH, Gandhi IC. Baclofen in trigeminal neuralgia – a clinical trial. *Indian J Dent Res* 1989; 1: 109–13.

Botulinum toxin
Argoff CE. Botulinum toxin. In: McCleane G and Smith (Eds), *Clinical management of bone and joint pain*. Haworth Press, Binghamton, USA, 2007.

Luvisetto S, Marinelli S, Cobianchi S, Pavone F. Anti-allodynic efficacy of botulinum neurotoxin A in a model of neuropathic pain. *Neuroscience* 2007; 145: 1–4.

Mahowald ML, Singh JA, Dykstra D. Long term effects of intra-articular botulinum toxin A for refractory joint pain. *Neurotox Res* 2006; 9: 179–88.

Placzek R, Drescher W, Deuretzbacher G et al. Treatment of chronic radial epicondylitis with botulinum toxin A. A double-blind, placebo-controlled, randomized multicenter study. *J Bone Joint Surg Am* 2007; 89: 255–60.

Qerama E, Fuglsang-Frederiksen A, Kasch H et al. A double-blind, controlled study of botulinum toxin A in chronic myofascial pain. *Neurology* 2006; 67: 241–5.

Tsai CP, Liu CY, Lin KP, Wang KC. Efficacy of botulinum toxin type A in the relief of carpal tunnel syndrome: a preliminary experience. *Clin Drug Investig* 2006; 26: 511–15.

Wong SM, Hui AC, Tong PY et al. Treatment of lateral epicondylitis with botulinum toxin: a randomized, double-blind, placebo controlled trail. *Ann Intern Med* 2005; 143: 793–7.

Yoon SJ, Ho J, Kang HY et al. Low-dose botulinum toxin type A for the treatment of refractory piriformis syndrome. *Pharmacotherapy* 2007; 27: 657–65.

Cimetidine

Yokoyama M, Aona H, Takeda A, Morita K. Cimetidine for chronic calcifying tendinitis of the shoulder. *Reg Anesth Pain Med* 2003; 28: 248–52.

Clonazepam

Bartusch SL, Sanders BJ, D'Alessio JG, Jernigan JR. Clonazepam for the treatment of lancinating phantom limb pain. *Clin J Pain* 1996; 12: 59–62.

Fishbain DA, Cutler RB, Rosomoff HL, Rosomoff RS. Clonazepam open clinical treatment trial for myofascial syndrome associated chronic pain. *Pain Med* 2000; 1: 332–9.

Gremeau-Richard C, Woda A, Navez ML et al. Topical clonazepam in stomatodynia: a randomised placebo-controlled study. *Pain* 2004; 108: 51–7.

Glucosamine

McAlindon TE, LaValley MP, Gulin JP, Felson DT. Glucosamine and chondroitin for treatment of osteoarthritis: a systematic quality assessment and meta-analysis. *JAMA* 2000; 283: 1469–75.

Poolsup N, Suthisisang C, Channark P, Kittikulsuth W. Glucosamine long-term treatment and the progression of knee osteoarthritis: systematic review of randomized controlled trials. *Ann Pharmacother* 2005; 39: 1080–7.

Towheed TE, Maxwell L, Anastassiades TP et al. Glucosamine therapy for treating osteoarthritis. *Cochrane Database Syst Rev* 2005; CD002946.

Hyaluronidase

Gourie-Devi M, Satish P. Intrathecal Hyaluronidase treatment of chronic spinal arachnoiditis of noninfective etiology. *Surg Neurol* 1984; 22: 231–4.

PART 2

CHAPTER 17
Neuropathic Pain

The treatment of neuropathic pain has progressed from the situation not so many years ago when there were few medicines with a specific neuropathic pain indication to the current state where that number has increased, although, particularly in the USA, those indications are for specific types of neuropathic pain rather than the entire spectrum of disorders where neuropathic pain is manifest. Therefore one has topical lidocaine, capsaicin, oral pregabalin, and gabapentin for postherpetic neuralgia but nothing with a specific indication for, to give an example, intercostal neuralgia or meralgia paresthetica.

In this chapter, a range of options for the treatment of neuropathic pain will be presented. Many of the options are "off-label," but hopefully from the following chapters readers will appreciate that while "off-label" there is a body of evidence that suggests both theoretical and practical reasons why they may have a pain-reducing effect. Naturally where such uses of medication are discussed the experiences and prejudices of the author will influence the options presented and those which are not mentioned. Hopefully the inclusion, or exclusion, of options is based on logic and practical clinical experience.

Neuropathic pain

Neuropathic pain is the result of injury or irritation of neural structures and is characterized by a number of distinct features:

Allodynia	Pain due to a stimulus that does not normally provoke pain
Dyesthesia	An unpleasant abnormal sensation, whether spontaneous or evoked
Paresthesia	An abnormal sensation, whether spontaneous or evoked
Hyperalgesia	An increased response to a stimulus which is normally painful
Hyperesthesia	Increased sensitivity to stimulation
Lancinating pain	Spontaneous or evoked pain with an "electric shock" like quality

Pain Management: Expanding the Pharmacological Options, Gary J. McCleane. © 2008 Blackwell Publishing, ISBN: 978-1-4051-7823-5.

Examples of conditions where neuropathic pain may be experienced		
• Trigeminal neuralgia	• Postherpetic neuralgia	• Intercostal neuritis
• Painful diabetic neuropathy	• Meralgia paresthetica	• Ilioinguinal neuralgia
• Genitofemoral neuralgia	• Carpal tunnel syndrome	• Ulnar neuritis
• Infra-orbital neuritis	• Supra-orbital neuritis	• Cervical radiculopathy
• HIV-associated neuropathy	• Lumbar radiculopathy	• Brachial neuritis
• Chemotherapy-related neuropathy	• Greater occipital	• Neuroma
• Femoral neuritis	neuritis	• Central poststroke pain

In any one individual some, or all, of these symptoms and signs may be present and the range of conditions that may give rise to neuropathic pain is large and diverse. In many cases a complex of neuropathic and non-neuropathic pain may co-exist, with the latter requiring different analgesic therapy to the former. Optimal control of the causative condition merits attention as well as that of the resultant pain. Therefore glycemic control in the diabetic patient with painful diabetic neuropathy or the relief of vascular occlusion in the patient with ischemic pain associated with peripheral vascular disease should accompany the direct attempts at relieving the resultant neuropathic pain.

"Novel" drug treatments for neuropathic pain

As well as knowledge of dosing of individual alternative drug therapies, an indication of duration of treatment before effect can be expected needs consideration. Should relief not be apparent after that period of time then the drug should be stopped. Even when relief is apparent, it should be continued only if the patient feels that the drug is improving the quality of life. Reduction of pain in the presence of intolerable drug-related side effects is no real benefit to the patient. Conversely, even a small reduction in pain in the absence of any side effects is often welcome (Table 17.1).

Active treatment of neuropathic pain can be either for long-term management or for acute flare-ups of pain. It is hoped that administration of medication on an ongoing basis may have a prophylactic effect in that it may curtail the frequency, magnitude, and duration of any flare-ups. When medication is used in the long term it should be chosen because of its tolerability being mindful that side effects of medication can be of slow onset and insidious as well as immediate and obvious.

In clinical practice referred, rather than radiated, pain is common. The referral of anginal pain to the jaw and left arm and that of diaphragmatic irritation to the shoulder tip are well known. Referred pain to the leg, for example, with facet joint problems or interspinous ligament irritation is also common. From a purely practical perspective the emphasis is on settling the condition which initiates the pain. Unfortunately this is not

Table 17.1 "Novel" drug treatments for neuropathic pain.

Drug	Dose	Time to effect
Topical		
Capsaicin 0.075% cream	4 times daily	4 weeks
Doxepin 5% cream	4 times daily	2–4 weeks
Lidocaine 5% patch	1–3 times daily	24 h
Oral		
L-Carnitine	500 mg twice daily	2 weeks
Baclofen*	10 mg thrice daily	24 h
Lamotrigine	50 mg daily increasing by 50 mg weekly to 300 mg a day	6 weeks
Duloxetine	60 mg at night	2 weeks
Ondansetron	4 mg thrice daily	24 h
Clonazepam	1.5 mg at night	24 h
Oxcarbazepine	150 mg 4 times daily	24 h
Intramuscular		
Phenytoin	400 mg	Hours
Fosphenytoin	500 PE units	Hours
Ondansetron	4 mg	Hours
Intravenous		
Phenytoin	1,000 mg over 24 h	24 h
Fosphenytoin	1,500 PE units over 24 h	24 h
Lidocaine	1,200 mg over 30 h	Up to 1 week
	or	
	1,000 mg over 8 h	Up to 1 week
Ondansetron	4 mg	Hours
Adenosine	50 mcg kg^{-1} over 60 min	24 h
Epidural		
Clonidine	150 mcg	2 days
Hyaluronidase**	3,000 IU	2 days

*For trigeminal neuralgia.
**Where neuropathic pain has resulted from postlaminectomy scar tissue/epidural fibrosis.

always successful. The treatment of referred pain is for all practical purposes the same as that for a radiated pain with AEDs, antidepressants, and membrane-stabilizing drugs all having a role.

Suggested algorithm

With the alternatives offered, if a single agent in a particular group fails to help, then another can be selected from the same group (Figure 17.1).

There are some circumstances where treatment with drugs not normally utilized for neuropathic pain treatment can indirectly reduce neuropathic pain. For example, the muscle relaxant baclofen can reduce the pain of

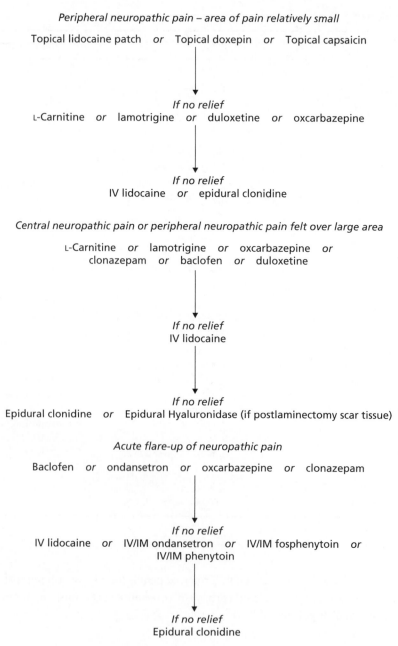

Peripheral neuropathic pain – area of pain relatively small

Topical lidocaine patch   *or*   Topical doxepin   *or*   Topical capsaicin

If no relief

L-Carnitine   *or*   lamotrigine   *or*   duloxetine   *or*   oxcarbazepine

If no relief

IV lidocaine   *or*   epidural clonidine

Central neuropathic pain or peripheral neuropathic pain felt over large area

L-Carnitine   *or*   lamotrigine   *or*   oxcarbazepine   *or*
clonazepam   *or*   baclofen   *or*   duloxetine

If no relief
IV lidocaine

If no relief

Epidural clonidine   *or*   Epidural Hyaluronidase (if postlaminectomy scar tissue)

Acute flare-up of neuropathic pain

Baclofen   *or*   ondansetron   *or*   oxcarbazepine   *or*   clonazepam

If no relief

IV lidocaine   *or*   IV/IM ondansetron   *or*   IV/IM fosphenytoin   *or*
IV/IM phenytoin

If no relief
Epidural clonidine

Figure 17.1 Suggested algorithm.

trigeminal neuralgia, while glyceryl trinitrate patches can be useful in the patient with ischemic neuritis caused by peripheral vascular disease or painful diabetic neuropathy where tissue ischemia can exacerbate neuropathic pain. The vasodilatory effects of nitrates can be used to maximize tissue perfusion and therefore indirectly reduce neuropathic pain.

CHAPTER 18

Complex Regional Pain Syndrome

Pharmacological management of this condition is difficult and all too many patients go on to develop chronic forms of the disorder. There is an impression that early intervention and active mobilization can improve the outlook, although the response to conventional pharmacological approaches is inconsistent and suboptimal.

Many will be more familiar with the other names that this condition has been labeled with. For example, among the previous labels were:

Reflex sympathetic dystrophy

Sudeks osteodystrophy

Shoulder hand syndrome

Algoneurodystrophy

The term "Complex regional pain syndrome" (CRPS) is preferred over reflex sympathetic dystrophy as patients may exhibit features that are either responsive to sympathetic blockade ("sympathetically maintained pain") or unresponsive ("sympathetic independent pain"). CRPS exists in two recognized forms. In CRPS type 1 (previously referred to as reflex sympathetic dystrophy) the patient may exhibit some or all of the following symptoms and signs:

- burning pain
- allodynia (mechanical and thermal)
- non-dermatomal pain
- swelling, which may be intermittent
- hyperhidrosis
- discoloration (often a dark bluish discoloration, which may be intermittent)
- localized osteoporosis
- hair loss
- contractures
- normal nerve function tests

Pain Management: Expanding the Pharmacological Options, Gary J. McCleane. © 2008 Blackwell Publishing, ISBN: 978-1-4051-7823-5.

In contrast, patients with CRPS type 2 exhibit the following features:
• burning pain
• dermatomal distribution of the pain
• abnormal nerve function tests

While CRPS type 1 is most often seen to affect the lower arm it can occur almost anywhere. Therefore it can be seen in the lower limb, face, breast, and even testicle, for example. A characteristic feature of CRPS type 1 is that the magnitude of the pain and the associated symptoms are often out of proportion with the initial injury. Therefore, what at the time seems a fairly mild soft tissue injury to the hand can progress to a disabling chronic affliction that leaves the limb virtually useless.

The pivotal role of the sympathetic nervous system is highlighted by what is standard treatment by many physicians for the condition. It is common practice for a stellate ganglion block or an intravenous (IV) regional sympathetic block to be undertaken for upper limb CRPS type 1. With the former technique a local anesthetic is injected around the stellate ganglion to cause temporary blockade of the sympathetic nerves traversing that structure, while with the latter technique a solution containing the sympathetic ganglion blocking agent guanethidine is injected into a vein in the exanguinated affected limb using a Bier's block technique. Where the pain is sympathetically maintained, prolonged relief can be produced, although a series of either blocks may be necessary. More recently, spinal cord stimulation has been used with effect, again with the aim of disrupting the sympathetic drive to the painful limb. Along with this interventional treatment a program of active mobilization is crucial.

However, access to this interventional therapy may be difficult and may take time. Any delay in receiving the treatment may have an impact of the prognosis. Therefore access to simpler pharmacological treatment that may prevent progression of the condition and impede the transition to chronicity is highly desirable.

Alternative pharmacological options for treatment of CRPS type 1

A range of potentially useful alternative therapies exist for the management of CRPS type 1 (Figure 18.1).

Topical options
• Capsaicin. It is well known that the repeated application of capsaicin can cause a reversible depletion of the neurotransmitter substance P and reduce the density of epidermal nerve fibers. Up to 4 weeks therapy may be necessary before effect is apparent. The discomfort of

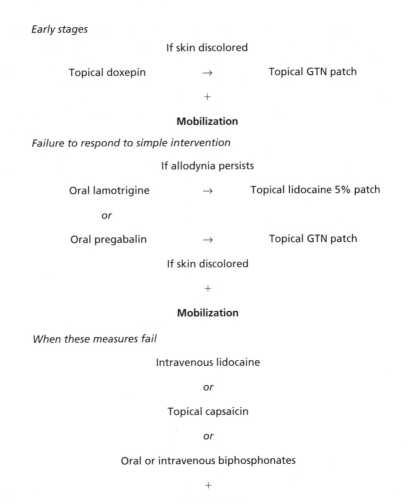

Early stages

If skin discolored

Topical doxepin   →   Topical GTN patch

+

Mobilization

Failure to respond to simple intervention

If allodynia persists

Oral lamotrigine   →   Topical lidocaine 5% patch

or

Oral pregabalin   →   Topical GTN patch

If skin discolored

+

Mobilization

When these measures fail

Intravenous lidocaine

or

Topical capsaicin

or

Oral or intravenous biphosphonates

+

Mobilization

Figure 18.1 Suggested treatment algorithm.

application can be reduced by co-administration of GTN. It may also enhance the effectiveness of the capsaicin.

- Doxepin. Peripheral, topical tricyclic antidepressant, in the form of doxepin 5%, can reduce pain by virtue of its effects on adenosine and opioid receptors and that on sodium channels. These structures are found in the periphery as well as in the central nervous system. Time to effect with treatment may be several weeks.
- Clonidine. Clonidine patches have been suggested as a therapy for CRPS type 1 and may interact with both peripheral and central α-adrenoreceptors
- Glyceryl trinitrate. While the major effect of topical GTN is on non-neuropathic pain it may also be useful for patients with CRPS type 1.

A prominent feature of CRPS type 1 is the dusky complexion of the skin that has a cyanotic appearance. The apparent reduction in tissue perfusion and oxygenation can do no good for skin, muscle, and nerve function in the affected area. This perfusion can be enhanced by peripheral nitrate application. Furthermore, allodynia is a feature of CRPS type 1. If the individual has an arthritic joint or tendonitis, for example, the presence of allodynia can exacerbate the pain from these conditions. The GTN can reduce that pain, and hence aid in overall pain management.

- Lidocaine. Topical lidocaine, in the form of the commercially available lidocaine 5% patch, may be useful in symptom alleviation. It can be particularly useful over allodynic areas where it can reduce the allodynia by virtue of the pharmacological action of lidocaine while the patch itself causes a physical barrier between the allodynic skin and any physical rubbing of that skin.
- Ketamine. Case report evidence suggests that topical ketamine ointment application can be effective during the acute phase of CRPS types 1 and 2 but also that it is ineffective when the process becomes chronic. It may achieve its effect by an action on peripheral glutamate receptors.

Oral

- Lamotrigine. Case report evidence suggests that lamotrigine can reduce the pain and other symptoms and signs of CRPS type 1. It tends to be less sedative than the other AEDs and is weight neutral. Slow dose titration is required to minimize the risk of skin rash.
- Gabapentin. While also being suggested by case reports it can cause sedation and weight gain.
- Pregabalin. Can also be useful in the treatment of CRPS type 1.
- Phenoxybenzamine. This orally active α-adrenoreceptor agonist can reduce CRPS type 1 pain but its use is often complicated by postural hypotension.
- Biphosphonates. Oral Alendronate has been shown to give marked relief in many patients with post-traumatic CRPS type 1.

Intravenous

- Lidocaine. Intravenous lidocaine infusions can reduce the pain, and in particular the allodynia associated with CRPS type 1. As previously described, an infusion administered over hours can reduce pain for weeks or even months. Tachyphylaxis does not seem to complicate treatment.
- Phentolamine. This drug is active on α-adrenoreceptors and is available in a parenteral formulation. When given by bolus IV injection a single dose can reduce CRPS pain for hours or even days. When given by IV infusion the relief can persist for weeks or even months. Intravenous phentolamine can cause hypotension consequent on peripheral

vasodilatation and this side effect can be reduced if the patient is preloaded with fluid prior to the commencement of phentolamine. A further side effect is that of palpitations. Even when phentolamine is diluted it can cause thrombophlebitis and so administration into a large vein is recommended while the use of a GTN patch above the infusion site can further reduce the risk of painful irritation of the vein.

- Ketamine. Intravenous infusion of ketamine at a dose of 40–80 mg day^{-1} for a 10-day period has been shown to reduce pain, improve mobility, and reduce autonomic dysregulation. The dose used is well below that which would be considered anesthetic.
- Biphosphonates. Intravenous pamidronate can reduce symptoms of CRPS type 1, although the response obtained is variable with some gaining good relief, others none.

Other treatments

Other treatment modalities have been mentioned for CRPS type 1 treatment but as yet have not become mainstream. These treatments include:

- Hyperbaric oxygen. Repetitive treatment with hyperbaric oxygen may reduce swelling and pain and improve range of movement in joints.
- Systemic corticosteroids. Prolonged therapy may be needed and therefore the side effects of prolonged corticosteroid therapy may complicate treatment.
- Thalidomide.
- Memantine. This drug has an action on N-methyl-D-aspartate receptors in the central nervous system. In one case report an 8-week treatment with memantine significantly reduced the symptoms of CRPS type 1.

When the simpler pharmacological interventions fail then consideration should be given to stellate ganglion, lumbar sympathetic or IV regional sympathetic blockade, or in resistant cases spinal cord stimulation.

Since referral and access to these more invasive procedures can take time, other pharmacological trials of agents mentioned above should be undertaken.

CHAPTER 19

Joint Pain

Essentially the treatment of joint pain falls into two major categories; first, the treatment of that disease process which gives rise to the joint pain in the first place and second the analgesic treatment of the pain consequent on the underlying disease process. Clearly there may be times that these considerations overlap, but the major focus of this chapter is on providing alternatives for managing pain rather than on primary treatment of the causitative disease.

Current analgesic treatment of joint pain utilizes a small number of drug classes. Non-steroidal anti-inflammatories (NSAIDs), both oral and topical, acetaminophen, opioids (mild, moderate, and strong), and corticosteroids are all used with varying degrees of success. Given that a major cause of joint pain relates to joint degeneration, symptoms of which increase with advancing age, some anxiety must be present about using potent medications with real risk of adverse effects, such as NSAIDs and opioids, in a patient population least able to tolerate the side effects that may be produced. It is hoped that the alternatives provided offer a low-risk strategy for managing patients with mono- and polyarticular joint pain.

The first step will be to describe those drugs that can be used to treat joint pain, sub-divided into sections according to their mode of administration followed by suggestions about how they can be used in clinical practice.

Topical options (Figure 19.1(a))

Capsaicin
The knowledge that repeated application of capsaicin, an extract from the chili pepper, can cause pain reduction is old and well known. Capsaicin may achieve its analgesic effect by virtue of its effects on reversibly depleting substance P and by reducing the density of epidermal nerve fibers. This effect may take weeks to become maximal and usually the unpleasant discomfort of application reduces as time progresses. However, compliance is reduced

---

Pain Management: Expanding the Pharmacological Options, Gary J. McCleane. © 2008 Blackwell Publishing, ISBN: 978-1-4051-7823-5.

because many find the burning discomfort of application intolerable. Even when it has reduced with time, should the application be accidentally applied outside the normal zone of application, a recurrence of the worst excesses of application pain may recur. Intuitively one would expect it to work best where the distance from skin to joint is small. The discomfort of application can be reduced by adding glyceryl trinitrate to the capsaicin, as described in an earlier chapter.

Monoarticular options

Topical/transdermal

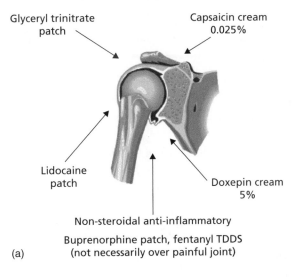

(a)

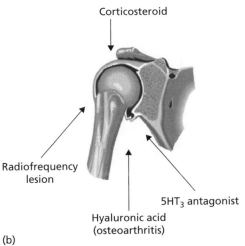

(b)

Figure 19.1 Suggested treatment algorithms for monoarticular pain. (a) Topical/transdermal options. (b) Intra-articular options.

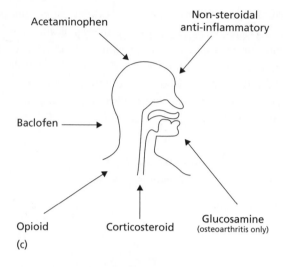

Acetaminophen

Non-steroidal
anti-inflammatory

Baclofen

Opioid

Corticosteroid

Glucosamine
(osteoarthritis only)

(c)

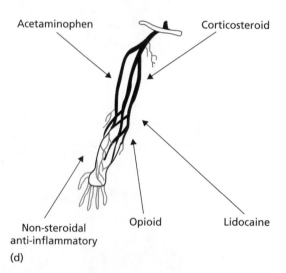

Acetaminophen

Corticosteroid

Non-steroidal
anti-inflammatory

Opioid

Lidocaine

(d)

Figure 19.1 (*Continued*). (c) Oral options. (d) Parenteral options.

Glyceryl trinitrate

When nitrates are applied topically they can reduce both pain and inflammation. This effect is maximal close to the site of administration. The most convenient form for application is that of a patch which is prepared for use in patients with angina. Unfortunately the dose available in these patches is greater than that needed to cause pain reduction and so the patch may need to be cut into segments. Therefore the impregnated membrane type rather than the depot with semipermeable membrane type patch is suggested. By using segments of the patch, coverage of a whole large joint or of several joints at a time can be achieved without too great a risk of nitrate-related side effects. Not unsurprisingly the most frequent side effect encountered is that of nitrate-related headache. Should this occur it would diminish shortly after patch removal. In contrast with its use in ischemic heart disease, tachyphylaxis does not seem to occur.

While glyceryl trinitrate ointment is available, it is hard to give a measured dose and it tends to stain clothes.

Lidocaine patch

Lidocaine 5% patch is available and is indicated for the treatment of post-herpetic neuralgia. However, it can be useful for the treatment of many other conditions, including joint pain. The dose of lidocaine absorbed from the patch, even if several are used at a time, is small and they can be used continually with a fresh patch, or patches being applied on a daily basis. They are reasonably large and so they can cover most joints. One issue is that there may be difficulty getting them to adhere to skin over a joint, especially if that joint is used extensively. Therefore, if being used on a knee, for example, they can be used along with a light-knee support to ensure that they remain closely applied to skin over that joint.

Doxepin

Historically among the first description of the use of an oral tricyclic antidepressant was in the treatment of joint pain. In practice this effect is small and it could be contended that the pain relief from tricyclic antidepressant use is outweighed by the side effects that frequently complicate the use. When a topical tricyclic antidepressant, such as doxepin, is used, that small amount of pain relief may be achieved without the complication of systemic tricyclic-related side effects.

Oral options (Figures 19.1(c) and 19.2(a))

Glucosamine

This dietary supplement can be remarkably effective in patients with osteoarthritis. While the bulk of the evidence that underpins its use refers to use in patients with osteoarthritis of the knee, from a clinical perspective those findings are replicated in other joints. Not only can pain be reduced, so too can joint stiffness. Time to effect may be measured in days to months. It is suggested in the literature that refers to knee osteoarthritis that the joint lining may increase in depth with sustained use and so it may be that glucosamine use can prevent osteoarthritis as well as actually treating it.

A number of other substances are often presented along with glucosamine. These include chondroitin and omega fish oils. The evidence base for additional benefit is probably strongest with chondroitin.

Baclofen

Although baclofen has absolutely no effect on joint pain as such, it can paradoxically be of help in patients with joint discomfort. When joint inflammation and pain occur, it is not unusual for that to be complicated by peri-articular muscle spasm. Relief of that spasm can increase joint range of movement and have a pain-relieving effect.

Intravenous options

Lidocaine

Intravenous lidocaine infusion not infrequently reduces joint pain. When joint inflammation occurs, the joint surface becomes almost allodynic. Therefore what would in the absence of joint pathology be normal joint movement triggers a pain response that inhibits further movement. It may well be that "sensitivity" that intravenous (IV) lidocaine infusions reduce. As previously described, the advantage of IV lidocaine is that an infusion over a matter of hours can give relief that persists for weeks and even months.

Intra-articular options (Figure 19(d))

A common intervention in those with joint pain is the intra-articular injection of corticosteroids. It is accepted that corticosteroids reduce inflammation and therefore pain. However, their pain-relieving effect may be produced by other pharmacological effects. It is now appreciated that corticosteroids specifically block C fibers, reduce ectopic discharge from damaged neurons, and have an effect on spinal dorsal horn cell function, and it may well be that these effects compound the pain relief produced by the reduction in inflammation.

Despite the often impressive results produced by intra-articular steroid injection, some anxieties exist about this therapy. First, the issue of how often such injections can be repeated before the harmful effects of corticosteroids outweigh the value of injection and second, worry about the total dose of steroid administered may reduce the number of joints that can be injected. One is therefore left with a therapeutic option of well-known efficacy but whose use both in terms of the number of joints that can be injected and the frequency of such injections is limited.

Fortunately some other intra-articular options exist.

5HT$_3$ antagonists

It has earlier been described how 5HT$_3$ antagonists can be used to treat fibromyalgia, irritable bowel syndrome, and neuropathic pain. It is now known that they can also be used by the intra-articular route and that the pain relief that is produced is at par with that produced by corticosteroid injection. When given into a joint, there is a clinical impression that they cause a flare of pain that can last for several days, before pain relief is produced. The benefit of use of this class of medication is that it is devoid of the risks associated with repeated corticosteroid injection.

Hyaluronic acid

Several hyaluronic acid preparations exist that are indicated for treatment of osteoarthritis of the knee – so called "viscosupplementation." These involve up to five separate intra-articular injections at weekly intervals. Not uncommonly, pain temporarily increases after the second or third injection, but when and if pain relief is produced it may persist for many months. It could be argued that if this treatment has an effect on the pain and stiffness associated with knee osteoarthritis, then it should have a similar effect when used in other joints for the same condition.

Biosynthetic options

Anakinra

Anakinra is a recombinant form of non-glycosylated human interleukin-1 receptor antagonist. This can have profound anti-inflammatory effects and can cause symptom improvement and suppression of cartilage and joint damage in rheumatoid arthritis. Furthermore, human study in patients with osteoarthritis has shown that its injection can cause symptom reduction that persists for up to 3 months.

Orgotein

This is a superoxide dimutase enzyme that acts as a powerful antioxidant. Oxygen free radicals act as potent promoters of inflammation by degrading cell walls and subsequently causing the release of lysosomal enzymes which promote the inflammatory process. Orgotein neutralizes these highly reactive and toxic oxygen-derived free radicals by catalyzing the conversion of two molecules of superoxide anion to one molecule of oxygen and one of hydrogen peroxide, eventually producing water. Orgotein may also inhibit phospholipase A2 activation and so impede release of prostaglandins and leukotrienes. In the synovial fluid of arthritic joints, superoxide radicals induce cartilage deterioration. Intra-articular injection of orgotein may inhibit this process. When used in patients with osteoarthritis, intra-articular injection may reduce symptoms for up to 3 months.

Octreotide

Octreotide is a somatostatin analog with a more favorable pharmacokinetic profile than its parent molecule and has been studied in a small number of patients with arthrosynovitis. When given by the intra-articular route in these patients, it can reduce pain and improve movement and function without significant systemic side effects.

Botulinum toxin

The use of botulinum toxin injections is well established in the treatment of muscle spasm. It may also be used by the peri- and intra-articular routes. Limited evidence from studies suggests that when used by intra-articular injection it may reduce joint pain by a direct analgesic effect.

Chloroquine

This drug has been used by the oral route for the treatment of a variety of rheumatologic conditions, although anxiety about potential adverse effects limit its use. There is also suggestion that when given by the intra-articular route it may reduce the symptoms of rheumatoid arthritis.

Opioids

It is now clear that opioid receptors exist in the periphery as well as in the central nervous system. Indeed, the concentration of opioid receptors increases in animal joints when inflammation is induced. Intra-articular opioids have been utilized for a number of years in the postoperative pain field after joint procedures with the suggestion that their effects are at least partially local ones, although systemic uptake and effect may be a welcome accompaniment.

Nerve blocks

Where a joint is supplied by a single nerve and that nerve is accessible, then perineural injection is possible. In most circumstances such injection will be with local anesthetic and corticosteroid. Unfortunately many joints have multiple nerves innervating them and so nerve blocks may be unhelpful or at best partially effective. While corticosteroids have a well-known anti-inflammatory effect, they may also suppress ectopic discharge from damaged neurons, have a weak local anesthetic effect, and suppress dorsal horn cell function, and these actions may contribute to their pain-relieving effect.

A good example of where a nerve block may significantly reduce joint pain is the suprascapular nerve block. The injectate is inserted into the suprascapular notch of the scapular and the block may help with a variety of shoulder joint and peri-articular conditions.

Why a proximally placed nerve block should help with a joint pain condition is interesting. The local anesthetic component of the injectate may temporarily anesthetize the joint, but it is common for the pain reduction to far outlive this local anesthetic effect. At least two possibilities exist. First, it is common for a depot steroid preparation to be used whose duration of effect lasts for weeks. If steroids have a weak local anesthetic effect, then this prolonged local anesthetic effect on the nerve may contribute to the reduction in joint pain. The second possibility is that as part of the inflammatory process substances are released in the joint that sensitize nerve endings and hence the supplying nerve and cause it to become overactive so that the joint surface becomes allodynic. The nerve block may reduce this induced allodynia.

Polyarticular options

All of the topical options listed above can be used on individual joints even when the pain affects multiple joints. Even with such polyarticular pain, patients will often identify one or a small number of joints as producing the worst pain: these can be targeted with the topical options, those agents with a more systemic effect being used for background pain relief for the other joints.

Polyarticular options

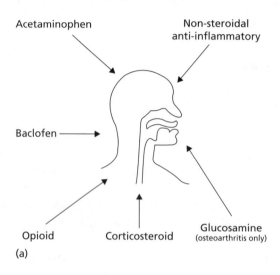

(a)

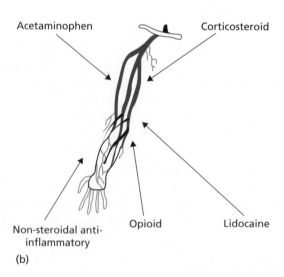

(b)

Figure 19.2 Polyarticular options. (a) Oral options. (b) Intravenous options.

CHAPTER 20

Fracture Pain

Conventional treatment of fracture pain revolves around the reduction of displaced bones, immobilization and utilization of analgesic medication. Opioids, non-steroidal anti-inflammatory drugs (NSAIDs), and acetaminophen are used, often successfully, in achieving the goal of pain relief.

Clearly, however, there will be circumstances where these drugs are either ineffective or where their use is contra-indicated. Perhaps some of the following options will offer a practical pharmacological alternative, always remembering that proper orthopedic management is paramount.

Pharmacological options

Inhalational

Nitrous oxide

Inhaled nitrous oxide has a long tradition in fracture pain management and is often used to facilitate patient transfer, fracture reduction, and splint application. However, those from an anesthesiological background will point out that the analgesia provided by nitrous oxide is inconsistent. Some patients derive quick and effective pain relief while others seem resistant to its use. Nitrous oxide should never be administered on its own but rather in conjunction with oxygen to avoid a potentially hypoxic mixture.

Topical skin

Glyceryl trinitrate

As previously described, topically applied nitrates, such as glyceryl trinitrate can have a local analgesic and anti-inflammatory effect. The only major side effect is nitrate headache, the risk of which can be reduced by using a smaller dose patch. While usually not on its own sufficient to reduce the pain of an acute fracture, it can be utilized in combination

Pain Management: Expanding the Pharmacological Options, Gary J. McCleane. © 2008
Blackwell Publishing, ISBN: 978-1-4051-7823-5.

with other treatment modalities or as a sole analgesic when a natural reduction in the fracture pain has begun.

Lidocaine 5% patch

Despite its indication for the treatment of postherpetic neuralgia, lidocaine patches can provide analgesia in a number of conditions. While probably inadequate to provide analgesia on its own after acute fracture, it becomes useful when used in combination with other analgesic interventions in the acute situation or on its own after the initial acute phase. Particularly it is useful in the treatment of pain from fractured ribs.

Fentanyl

Transdermal fentanyl can provide useful background analgesia. Each patch remains applied for 72 h during which a steady state for the drug is achieved.

Topical: mucous membrane

Diamorphine

Desirable characteristics of any analgesic used in fracture pain treatment are efficacy, speed of onset, and ease of administration. A widely used method of acute analgesic administration is by intramuscular injection of an opioid such as morphine. It could be well argued that an intravenous (IV) administration of that opioid would be more appropriate, but the reality is in clinical practice that intramuscular injection is more widely used and accepted by clinical staff than IV use. Despite which method is contemplated, some patients, and in particular children, dislike any form of injection. It is known that the nasal mucous membrane is a well-perfused structure and that a variety of drugs can be administered by application onto this membrane. Diamorphine is among the drugs known to be absorbed efficiently from mucous membrane and has been shown to be a useful tool in fracture analgesic therapy.

Fentanyl

While transdermal fentanyl has use as a background treatment of fracture pain, it is unlikely to provide much relief when movement of a fracture is likely as during patient transfer or splint application. In these circumstances fentanyl lozenges/lollipops can provide rapid onset, intense analgesia.

Oral

Non-steroidal anti-inflammatory drugs

NSAID is one of the primary building blocks of fracture pain management. It is used either alone, or often with added value when used in combination with other agents. Selection of which NSAID to use is largely based on personal preference and experience.

Opioids

Opioid analgesics have much merit in the short-term management of fractures but are better at reducing the background pain that accompanies a fracture rather than the acute pain associated with movement. Given their propensity to induce constipation, prophylactic measures to prevent this eventuality are advisable. Those analgesics that contain codeine are not universally effective as a proportion of the population lack the cytochrome P450 enzyme necessary to convert codeine to morphine and hence to activate it. The same difficulty does not occur with dihydrocodeine or tramadol.

For more severe pain strong opioids may be necessary. For the most acute situations immediate release strong opioids should be selected while for less acute situations sustained release preparations supplemented by immediate release for breakthrough pain.

Acetaminophen

When used at appropriate doses, oral acetaminophen is an effective analgesic with a relatively benign side effect profile. Only in overdose does it become less safe. Regular dosing with acetaminophen, often with an NSAID is an effective treatment that should be instituted early and only supplemented with other agents or techniques if therapeutic failure occurs.

Muscle relaxants

Skeletal muscle relaxants have no analgesic effect for pure bone fracture pain. However, muscle spasm is a frequent accompaniment of any fracture, can be painful by itself, but most importantly increases fracture pain by compounding the mal-alignment of fractured bone. Fracture reduction and stabilization may by themselves reduce or remove muscle spasm, but where it remains troublesome, a skeletal muscle relaxant drug may be indicated. Baclofen has a fairly rapid onset of action and a favorable side effect profile and can be used in adults at a dose of 15–60 mg daily in three divided doses. Where muscle spasm becomes chronic, then other agents such as dantrolene or tizanadine may be considered. Alternatively, if the spasm is confined to a well-defined muscle or muscle group, then botulinum toxin injection may become an option.

Parenteral

Opioids

Parenteral administration of strong opioids is appropriate in the acute situation after fracture, when flare-ups of pain are expected (movement, splint application, etc.) and in the face of failure with other analgesic interventions. Parenteral morphine or oxycodone may be preferable to shorter-acting opiates such as meperidine.

Acetaminophen

The recent availability of an IV formulation of acetaminophen offers a new alternative to fracture pain management. A 1 g infusion of acetaminophen has comparable analgesic effect to 10 mg morphine. Indeed, parenteral acetaminophen may be preferable to parenteral strong opioid as the risks of nausea, sedation, and respiratory depression are avoided.

Ketamine

The intramuscular or IV administration of ketamine at correct doses is associated with pain relief which can be profound. At greater doses it becomes anesthetic. Consequently, ketamine can be used to facilitate fracture reduction and splint application.

Ketamine has some merit in that it maintains blood pressure which contrasts it with other potentially anesthetic agents. However, excess salivation can occur and patients may experience unpleasant dreams and hallucinations when it is used, and so its utility is limited.

Lidocaine

Anecdotal evidence suggests that the IV administration of lidocaine can have a significant analgesic effect with a variety of fractures and most particularly with rib fractures. Indeed the pain relief apparent after IV lidocaine can far outlast the half-life of the drug. Lidocaine infusion is not associated with side effects of opioids such as nausea, sedation, or respiratory depression and even cardiovascular side effects which one would intuitively associate with lidocaine use are rare. Clinically doses of 1,000–1,200 mg over a 24-h period can be used with dose adjustment depending on the size, age, and health status of the patient.

Propofol

This drug is used in anesthesiological practice to achieve induction of anesthesia. In this use it is given intravenously and the dose titrated to effect. This usually requires administration at least $2 \, \text{mg kg}^{-1}$ of the drug. When it is used at much lower doses, $0.5–0.75 \, \text{mg kg}^{-1}$, it can reduce pain and have an amnesic effect without inducing anesthesia and can be used to allow a fracture to be reduced, an external splint applied or the patient moved without undue discomfort. It has a short duration of effect and therefore fairly rapid return to a pre-injection state is usually observed.

Perineural

Nerve blocks

Single shot nerve blocks are of little value in all but the most acute of situations where they may reduce the worst excesses of fracture pain until more definitive treatment is instituted. Examples of where these single shot nerve blocks may be of value include femoral or "three-in-one" blocks for femoral fractures, intercostal or paravertebral blocks for rib fractures, and suprascapular nerve blocks for upper humeral fractures and shoulder dislocations. A longer-lasting local anesthetic such as bupivicaine is preferable to those with less prolonged durations of effect.

Nerve blocks can be used to allow fracture manipulation and splint application: brachial plexus block being used for upper limb fracture manipulation, femoral nerve block for femoral fracture interventions.

A further technique which can allow manipulation or intervention on upper limb fractures is the IV regional block ("Bier's Block") where lidocaine is given intravenously on the affected side after a cuff is inflated above systolic pressure on that limb proximally. Good practice suggests that in fact a double cuff is used to minimize the risk of systemic leakage of the lidocaine.

A more localized technique is the hematoma block, usually used for distal forearm fractures, where local anesthetic is injected into the fracture hematoma.

Epidurals

The major utilization of epidurally administered drugs is in the management of rib fractures and chest trauma. Given that no operated intervention is normally possible for rib fractures, pain relief is a fundamental goal in rib fracture management.

Treatment of specific fractures

Rib fractures

Even isolated rib fractures can be the cause of morbidity and mortality. The impairment of respiratory function that is the almost inevitable consequence of the pain associated with a rib fracture can be enough to induce respiratory failure in those with pre-existent respiratory disease. When these fractures are multiple, even those with previous good health can be pushed into respiratory failure. When major trauma is involved, rib fractures may be associated with lung contusion and injury which increases the risk of complications.

By their nature, rib fractures are not normally amenable to surgical fixation. The basis of treatment is therefore adequate pain relief. The full range of treatment options outlined above can be utilized. Because of the close relationship between rib fractures and respiratory function, the adequacy of treatment can be measured by undertaking simple respiratory tests. For example, when the effect of IV fentanyl is compared with the extradural infusion of the same dose of fentanyl, the effect can be compared by measuring vital capacity, $PaCO_2$, PaO_2, SaO_2, and so on. When this is done, extradural infusion of fentanyl appears to improve these parameters more so than IV infusion of the same dose.

A variety of specific local anesthetic techniques have gained popularity in the management of rib fracture pain. Their principal appeal is that they allow a greater depth of inspiration and active events such as coughing to be undertaken in a more normal fashion. In contrast to the use of strong opioids, this effect is produced without significant sedation or respiratory depression. While single shot blocking procedures, such as the intercostal nerve block, often produce pain relief, their duration of effect is only as long as the duration of action of the local anesthetic used. Therefore, infusion techniques are more appropriate.

One such technique is the intrapleural infusion of a local anesthetic such as bupivicaine. An epidural type catheter is inserted intercostally and bupivicaine infused.

A second local anesthetic technique involves the insertion of a catheter into the paravertebral space and the infusion of a local anesthetic with the most popular choice being bupivicaine. When rib fractures are unilateral this is a viable option. When they are bilateral it is not.

Perhaps the most common local anesthetic intervention is the thoracic epidural infusion. Utilization of this technique has become the norm when simple interventions fail and when signs of respiratory impairment become apparent. In many instances the insertion of a thoracic epidural catheter and the infusion of a local anesthetic, usually in combination with an opioid, can prevent the need to institute mechanical ventilation because of the respiratory impairment caused by the pain from the fractured ribs. Even when ventilation is required, a thoracic epidural allows a lower level of sedation to be used and aids in weaning from ventilation.

A less common local anesthetic intervention is the IV infusion of lidocaine. When lidocaine is given intravenously, pain relief is often produced without the expected complication of numbness. Cardiovascular side effects are in reality rare. Clinical practice suggests that in a healthy adult a dose of 1,000 mg of lidocaine infused over 24 h has a reasonable chance of producing pain relief.

In the case of a sternal, as opposed to rib fracture, an additional local anesthetic technique exists. A catheter can be inserted sub-periosteally in the sternum, close to the fracture and local anesthetic, with or without an opioid infused (see Figure 20.1).

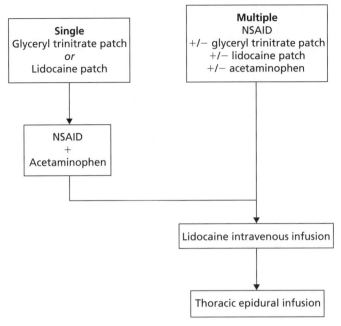

Figure 20.1 Treatment of rib fractures.

Femoral fractures

It goes without saying that the pain from a major long bone fracture is severe and that simple analgesic techniques are rarely sufficient to obtund this pain. Fortunately the nerve supply to the upper femur is relatively easily accessed and therefore amenable to local anesthetic techniques. Deposition of long-lasting local anesthetic, such as bupivicaine, around the femoral nerve can give partial relief. When a larger volume is used, a so-called "three-in-one block" can be achieved – the femoral, lateral cutaneous, and quadratus femoris nerves are all blocked. Alternatively a fascia iliaca compartment block can be used.

Vertebral collapse fractures

In the fit and healthy, considerable force is required to fracture a vertebra (Table 20.1). In the patient with osteoporosis this can happen with forces that would otherwise be inconsequential. As with any fracture, immediate pain is normal after the fracture. What is more problematical is that pain can be a long-term consequence of such a fracture. When a vertebral body is traumatized to the extent that fracture occurs, its physical shape is often altered. A vertebral body exists in a dynamic structure/function relationship to its surrounding structures and so with a change in shape, its architectural relationships change as well. The list of alterations that can occur is long (Figure 20.2).

Table 20.1 Alternatives for the treatment of vertebral fracture pain (medium and long term).

Interspinous ligament	*Muscle spasm*
NSAID	Baclofen
Capsaicin	Methocarbamol
GTN patch	Cyclobenzaprine
Lidocaine patch	Dantrolene
Topical doxepin cream	NSAID
Local anesthetic/steroid injection	Botulinum toxin
$5HT_3$ antagonist injection	*Facet Joint pain*
Radiated/Referred pain	NSAID
Pregabalin	Capsaicin
Gabapentin	Lidocaine patch
Lamotrigine	Corticosteroid joint injection
Oxcarbazepine	$5HT_3$ antagonist injection
Carbamazepine	Radiofrequency lesioning
Tricyclic antidepressant	Epidural corticosteroid injection

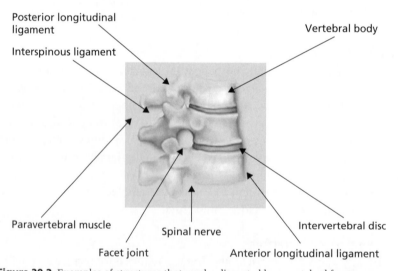

Posterior longitudinal ligament

Interspinous ligament

Vertebral body

Paravertebral muscle

Spinal nerve

Intervertebral disc

Facet joint

Anterior longitudinal ligament

Figure 20.2 Examples of structures that can be disrupted by a vertebral fracture.

Each one of these structures can give rise to pain. For example, unnatural stresses on an interspinous ligament can give rise to localized pain over the ligament with pain worse on back flexion. On occasions this is accompanied by a referred pain in the dermatomal distribution of the spinal nerves arising at that level. Being a mid-line structure, these ligaments often give rise to referred pain which is bilaterally experienced. More problematical is the question of the pain that arises from structures such as the anterior longitudinal ligament that has a sympathetic innervation and elements of the disc margin that have both somatic and sympathetic innervation. The quality and distribution of the pain arising from disruption of these structures is poorly defined.

When nerve impingement occurs, a radiated neuropathic pain is the consequence and is suggested by the usually diagnostic symptoms and signs of neuropathic pain (e.g., paresthesia, numbness, allodynia, and lancinating pain). Therefore, adequate treatment of the longer-term pain that can occur with a vertebral collapse fracture requires a diagnosis as to which structure, or structures, are giving rise to the pain. Only then can there be significant hope of good quality pain relief.

CHAPTER 21

Postoperative Pain

It is probably fair to say that the management of postoperative pain has more uniformity and consistency than the treatment of most other pain-related conditions. The use of opioids, non-steroidal anti-inflammatory drugs (NSAIDs), acetaminophen, and local anesthetics form the backbone of treatment and are often highly effective in reducing pain. With the passage of time new ways of administering each drug has further improved our ability to reduce postoperative pain. We can now, for example, give acetaminophen intravenously, local anesthetic around the wound, and opioid by the intrathecal route. But, on occasions, patients still suffer undue postoperative pain either because of resistance to the analgesics used or because these analgesics cannot be used because of contraindications or undue side effects.

The following options may offer an alternative should our normal interventions fail.

Clonidine

This α-adrenoreceptor agonist is available in topical, oral, and injectable formulations. The epidural and intrathecal use of clonidine is firmly established in postoperative pain management where its use is associated with enhanced analgesia and decreased opioid requirements in the postoperative phase. Isolated studies also suggest other analgesic uses for this medication. When used orally it can cause sedation, which may be of value when used as a premedicant drug, and reduce postoperative pain. When added to local anesthetics and infiltrated into postoperative wounds, the addition of the clonidine can significantly prolong the duration of effect of the local anesthetic. This effect can be achieved with doses far below that which would be needed to cause hypotension or sedation.

Pain Management: Expanding the Pharmacological Options, Gary J. McCleane. © 2008
Blackwell Publishing, ISBN: 978-1-4051-7823-5.

Dexamethasone

The use of dexamethasone as an antiemetic in the postoperative phase is well described. In addition, it is widely accepted that use of corticosteroids can reduce the pain after tonsillectomy and tooth extraction. Others report that when dexamethasone is used intravenously it can not only reduce the nausea often experienced after intrathecal opioid use but also improve the quality of pain relief produced by that intrathecal opioid. Conversely, when corticosteroid is used along with a local anesthetic in a nerve block for post-operative pain, the duration and quality of pain relief produced is no different from that produced by the nerve block alone. This contrasts to the clinical impression that addition of corticosteroid to local anesthetic for use in a nerve block for many chronic pain conditions does have a significant effect on the quality and duration of the relief provided by that intervention.

In those circumstances where the like of dexamethasone does reduce postoperative pain it may be because of a number of effects. First, corticosteroids reduce inflammation and swelling. Second, they can have a weak local anesthetic effect and reduce the ectopic discharge from damaged neurons, and third, they can stabilize otherwise overactive spinal dorsal horn cells.

Gabapentinoids

The gabapentinoids, gabapentin, and pregabalin exert their analgesic effect by interaction with the α–$\delta 2$ sub-unit of the calcium channel and are known to have an anti-allodynic and anti-hyperalgesic effect when used in the treatment of neuropathic pain. It is now known that these drugs can also reduce postoperative pain, reduce postoperative opioid requirement, and consequently reduce opioid-related side effects. Interestingly, the current evidence would suggest that the opioid-sparing effect of gabapentin is not dependent on the dose of gabapentin used.

Ketamine

Ketamine has long been available for anesthesiological use. Traditionally it was used to induce anesthesia, but when used at the doses required for this effect its use was often complicated by emergence delirium. Since then it has become firmly established as an adjunct to postoperative analgesia. Substantial evidence now exists that when it is administered at a low dose, that is well below that required to induce anesthesia, postoperative opioid requirements are reduced, pain control improved, and the incidence of postoperative nausea and vomiting also reduced, all in the absence of significant ketamine-related side effects.

Lidocaine

Intravenous

The first report of the use of an intravenous (IV) local anesthetic was in the management of burns pain while that of lidocaine dates back to 1961 and describes use in postoperative pain management. Since that time a variety of reports have suggested that IV lidocaine infusion reduces postoperative pain and opioid consumption, shortens hospital stay, quickens mobilization, and in the case of use after major colorectal surgery, shortens the time to first passage of a bowel motion. Infusions are generally commenced during the operative intervention and continued for 24 h after. The pain relief after such short-term infusions often persists for many days and not just for that period where the drug has a significant plasma concentration.

Topical

The lidocaine 5% patch contains approximately 700 mg of the drug, of which only a small fraction is released. It has an indication for the treatment of postherpetic neuralgia. In many surgical operations, a significant proportion of the pain produced is due to the surgical trauma to the skin. This is confirmed by the good quality pain reduction seen when the skin is infiltrated with local anesthetic at the end of the procedure. However, currently available local anesthetics have a relatively short duration of action and so that good quality pain relief after their use may only last for a matter of hours. It would seem obvious that the topical application of a local anesthetic containing preparation over the postoperative wound which allows administration of that local anesthetic for a prolonged period (with the patch being changed every 24 h until the pain naturally subsides) would improve the quality of postoperative pain relief. Lidocaine 5% patch may represent a mechanism for achieving this goal. While there are no studies or even case reports to add weight to this supposition, in my institution we have been using topical lidocaine 5% patches over postoperative wounds with to us what is obvious success. Whether the 5% formulation is the correct dosing to achieve maximal effect is open to speculation.

Magnesium

Conflicting results have been reported when magnesium is administered for postoperative pain. When used intravenously many of these reports show no improvement in postoperative pain, whereas isolated reports of epidural use suggest that when used by this route opioid requirements during the postoperative phase are reduced. In chronic pain practice, magnesium infusion can reduce pain and more particularly chronic muscle spasm and it may be that any effect seen in the postoperative phase is due to reduced muscle tone around the postoperative wound with a consequent indirect reduction in wound pain rather than a direct analgesic effect.

Nitrates

Topically applied nitrates can reduce both pain and inflammation. While this effect is maximal locally, some studies also suggest that nitrates can have an opioid-potentiating effect when the nitrate is used in doses sufficient to achieve systemic levels.

   Glyceryl trinitrate patch or patches can be applied close to the operative wound for localized pain relief. Additional potential benefit includes increased perfusion of the wound area which may have an effect on wound healing and a systemic absorption causing a cardioprotective effect. Nitrate patches come into their own in particular circumstances:

1 When non-steroidal anti-inflammatories are contraindicated because of renal, cardiovascular, gastrointestinal, or hematological disease; because they have a different mode of action to non-steroidal anti-inflammatories, they can also be used as a complement to NSAID-associated analgesia.

2 As "step-down" analgesia for example when an epidural is discontinued. The major drawback to nitrate use is nitrate headache which can be of a severity to cause discontinuation. From a practical perspective those nitrate patches which are of the drug-impregnated membrane type can be cut into segments and placed around the wound to minimize the total nitrate dose used.

Non-steroidal anti-inflammatories

Oral and parenteral non-steroidal anti-inflammatories are clearly widely used in postoperative pain management. What is less well known is that they can also be infiltrated or infused into postoperative wounds. When used in this fashion they can reduce pain and the dose requirements of opioid analgesics to a greater extent than when a similar dose is used systemically.

Topical local anesthetics

Several non-patch topical local anesthetic formulations are available and are used to reduce the pain of venipuncture. These preparations include

EMLA® (eutectic mixture of local anesthetics) cream which contains prilocaine and lidocaine and amethocaine gel. These can be used in the postoperative phase for reducing the pain associated with the like of circumcision.

Conclusion

Postoperative pain is predictable both in its nature, location, and possibly duration. It has therefore been possible to institute treatment protocols for its management, which are effective in the majority of cases. On those occasions when the usual medications are ineffective, or where it is not possible to use them because of patient intolerance or contraindication, some of the above alternatives may be usefully applied. Those options listed above fall into two categories. First, there are those which have been reported to be effective but whose use is as yet not supported by a vast weight of evidence and second, those whose use is anecdotal. With some, such as nitrate and lidocaine patches, we have found to be of considerable value and their risk in terms of side effects to be minimal.

CHAPTER 22
Fibromyalgia

Pain is a prominent symptom in the condition known as fibromyalgia. Along with sleep and mood disturbance, bladder and bowel symptoms the pain of fibromyalgia represents a significant treatment challenge to the physician. Widespread muscle tenderness may co-exist with joint pain and even symptoms suggestive of neuropathic pain, such as paresthesia and tingling. The pain of this condition seems to respond poorly to conventional analgesic therapy and even the non-steroidal anti-inflammatories are relatively ineffective. Perhaps the only major exception is in the case of tramadol which can have a pain-reducing effect.

Conventional pain therapy for the patient with fibromyalgia is with the tricyclic antidepressant drugs, even if none has a specific fibromyalgia indication. More recently the Selective Serotonin Reuptake Inhibitors (SSRIs) have gained popularity, although the evidence of a pain-reducing effect is less impressive than that with the tricyclics. The suggestion is that the tricyclics can reduce pain and muscle spasm while promoting a more regular sleep pattern with any antidepressant effect being of value in elevating the patient's mood.

To many physicians this is the limit of the treatment options that they utilize. Suggestions to take tricyclics, accompanied by advice to mobilize, are followed by early discharge from care. It could be argued that treatment of a more efficacious nature is and should be available to patients with fibromyalgia.

It should not be assumed that tricyclic antidepressants or indeed opioid analgesics are always pain relievers. In the case of tricyclic antidepressants, a number of animal studies suggest that their use can be complicated by paradoxical pain. Specifically, when given to animals with an induced neuropathic pain, the tricyclic reduces the neuropathic pain on the side of neural injury, but can make the contralateral, and non-injured, side allodynic. In the case of opioids, both animal and human evidence shows that sustained opioid use can cause hyperesthesia and

Pain Management: Expanding the Pharmacological Options, Gary J. McCleane. © 2008 Blackwell Publishing, ISBN: 978-1-4051-7823-5.

muscle spasm. The human relevance of such paradoxical pain caused by the use of members of these two drug classes remains to be firmly established, but emphasizes that any use of these drugs should be followed by careful assessment of both their positive and negative effects with sustained use only taking place if in the patients' judgment their use is helpful. There should be no place for ongoing treatment with these drugs if no discernable benefit accrues from their use.

Fibromyalgia pain

Classically the pain associated with fibromyalgia is muscle based and accompanied by identifiable areas of muscle tenderness. Indeed, the diagnosis is made based on the presence of a certain number of these trigger spots. In practice, patients also often complain of joint pain, skin sensitivity, tingling, and paresthesia as well as symptoms associated with irritable bowel syndrome and interstitial cystitis which are a frequent accompaniment. To an extent these pain symptoms represent the classic fibromyalgia picture with the condition being indivisibly linked to these types of pain. But patients with fibromyalgia also suffer pain resulting from, for example, trauma, surgical intervention, and degenerative disease. Therefore, one cannot assume that when confronted with a patient with known fibromyalgia that all pain they develop must be due to that fibromyalgia. It may be that the fibromyalgia influences, and usually magnifies pain from any source, but in circumstances where a fibromyalgia patient experiences pain which is exaggerated by the fibromyalgia but not caused by it, then the emphasis must be on the management of the initiating cause. Therefore, in the patient with fibromyalgia who presents with, for example, joint pain, a diagnostic process must be undertaken to identify the cause of the joint pain and not an assumption made that it must be caused by fibromyalgia. Furthermore, there is the clinical impression that fibromyalgia may be triggered by trauma, neuropathic pain, severe emotional upset, and the like and the consequences of these provocating conditions co-exist with the resultant fibromyalgia.

The treatment of fibromyalgia pain divides, therefore, into three categories:

1 The treatment of the pain directly attributable to the fibromyalgia.
2 The treatment of those associated non-pain symptoms that are often apparent and which may directly, or indirectly, influence fibromyalgia pain.
3 Treatment of non-fibromyalgia pain provoking conditions which may themselves be influenced by the fibromyalgia.

Therefore, when assessment of a patient with fibromyalgia is undertaken, the types of pain relief that may be appropriately suggested may include standard fibromyalgia pain treatment and treatments for individual non-fibromyalgia pain conditions. This creates a rather confusing situation. Non-steroidal anti-inflammatory drugs have no proven benefit in the analgesic management of fibromyalgia. However, the fibromyalgia patient with painful osteoarthritis may gain relief when such non-steroidals are used. Therefore, while one could say that non-steroidal anti-inflammatory drugs do not help fibromyalgia pain, they may still help patients with fibromyalgia.

Because fibromyalgia encompasses a complex of symptoms the concentration on one may not be of overall benefit if it exacerbates other features of the condition. For example, opioid analgesics may provide a degree of pain relief but may worsen the symptoms of irritable bowel syndrome to the extent that the adverse effects of their use outweigh any analgesic benefit. Therefore, when an analgesic treatment plan is constructed, it must be influenced not only by that pain with which the patient presents, but also by those other non-pain symptoms that form part of that patient's fibromyalgia and by co-existing conditions and drug therapy.

Pain therapies

A variety of pain therapies will be outlined and indications given for which particular types of fibromyalgia pain they are superior for and how they may be used in practical clinical management. They are not laid out in any order of superiority, but rather alphabetically.

$5HT_3$ antagonist

Conventionally used in the treatment and prevention of postoperative and cancer chemotherapy associated nausea and vomiting, the $5HT_3$ antagonists may be utilized in a number of ways in the fibromyalgia patient:

- Oral $5HT_3$ antagonists such as tropisetron, granisetron, and ondansetron can be used either as background analgesic maintenance therapy or when quick pain relief is required during a flare-up of the condition. They can be given by the oral and parenteral route.
- The $5HT_3$ antagonist allosetron has a specific indication in the USA for diarrhea preponderant irritable bowel syndrome in female patients and it may be that the other $5HT_3$ antagonists share this property.
- Tender points in muscles and painful joints can be injected with $5HT_3$ antagonists and when used in this fashion the relief apparent is comparable to that obtained by corticosteroid injection.

Unfortunately $5HT_3$ antagonists are expensive, and the cost implications of long-term use may be prohibitive. Serious adverse effects with their use are infrequent. Headache and constipation are relatively common, while isolated reports of ischemic colitis with allosetron use have been made. There may be a bell-shaped dose–response curve with $5HT_3$ antagonists with high doses being rewarded with less pain relief than moderate doses.

L-Carnitine

Both animal and human studies have shown that carnitine can reduce neuropathic pain and in particular that associated with cancer chemotherapy. It can also have a useful effect in patient with fibromyalgia. In the UK carnitine is sold in health food shops and has a suggested indication of weight loss (it has an effect on fat metabolism) and depression. Many patients like the concept of using something that is freely available over the counter and perceive that type of availability as indicating safety with use. We know that carnitine has an effect of glutamate receptors and this is probably what endows it with pain-relieving properties. Side effects with use are few and any antidepressant effect in a patient group in whom depression is a frequent accompaniment is welcome. A number of the drugs used conventionally in fibromyalgia treatment, such as the tricyclic antidepressants, and certain anti-epileptics are known to cause weight gain, so the propensity of carnitine to achieve weight loss may again be welcome.

Clonazepam

Sleep disturbance is a major problem in patients with fibromyalgia. Tricyclics are often initiated as much to regularize sleep patterns as to reduce pain. Clonazepam, a long-acting benzodiazepine, can be a useful alternative to a tricyclic. It combines analgesic, antispasmodic, and anxiolytic properties with its hypnotic effects. Morning "hangover" is a real possibility after dosing the previous evening and may require careful manipulation of dose to minimize this troublesome side effect. That said, clonazepam is a useful drug particularly as its major effects mirror what is problematical in the fibromyalgia patient.

Clonidine

While the side effects of oral clonidine limit its use, caudal epidural clonidine can give useful relief that can persist for up to 2 months. Caudal epidural injections can be relatively painful to receive but have the advantage of having minimal risk of inadvertent dural puncture. On the other hand, the caudal hiatus can be relatively difficult to locate in some individuals.

Doxepin

While the use of oral tricyclic antidepressants in patients with fibromyalgia is widespread, use of the topical formulations of these drugs, of which doxepin is the most readily available, is less common. Since the tricyclics may achieve pain relief by both peripheral and central modes of action, the topical, peripheral use of these drugs can achieve pain relief without the side effects associated with the systemic use of these drugs. Clearly fibromyalgia is a condition where pain is widespread and the extensive use of a topical tricyclic would be associated with significant systemic uptake and side effects, patients with fibromyalgia often complain of pain that is worse in certain locations and these can be therapeutically targeted with a topical tricyclic antidepressant such as doxepin.

Duloxetine

While the tricyclics have a long pedigree of use in patients with fibromyalgia, there is no doubt that their use is often complicated with troubling side effects. Furthermore, when pain relief is apparent, it is rarely of dramatic proportions. The advent of the serotonin norepinephrine reuptake inhibitors (SNRIs), such as duloxetine, offers the prospect of pain relief and improvement of mood but with less frequent side effects than that with the tricyclics. It could be argued, therefore, that they should be used in preference to the tricyclics. Further, since the SSRIs have marked antidepressant effects but only weak analgesic actions, it is probably fair to say that the SNRIs should be used in preference to the SSRIs. Unfortunately, if a tricyclic or SSRI is discontinued and an SNRI commenced, the withdrawal of the original antidepressant can precipitate a withdrawal type reaction which can manifest itself as a severe headache accompanied by nausea, anxiety, and an increase in pain. That said, in a significant proportion of patients the change from a tricyclic or SSRI to an SNRI is rewarded either by an improvement in pain relief or by a lessening in drug-related side effects. In some patients both outcomes are achieved.

Gabapentinoids

Both pregabalin and gabapentin can reduce fibromyalgia pain. When pregabalin is used, rapid titration is possible. The gabapentinoids can reduce all modalities of fibromyalgia pain and not just that which has a neuropathic element. Because pregabalin can be quickly titrated, it can be used as a short-term treatment for flare-ups of fibromyalgia pain.

Lamotrigine

One could argue about which anti-epileptic drug is the most efficient at reducing fibromyalgia pain. Lamotrigine is particularly effective when used for the neuropathic type symptoms that can occur in patients with fibromyalgia. Its advantages, apart from its analgesic effectiveness, include the fact that it has no effect on the patients' weight, in contrast to many other anti-epileptics, the lack of sedation associated with use and its safety in pregnancy. Skin rash is the most frequent adverse effect with use and its incidence can be lessened by a slow escalation of lamotrigine dose.

Lidocaine: intravenous

The intravenous (IV) infusion of lidocaine can produce pain relief that persists for much longer than the infusion period or the useful plasma half-life of the drug. Therefore, an infusion given over 30h, for example, can be rewarded with pain relief that persists for weeks, and even months. The advantage of this form of therapy is that during the period of pain relief, the patient can reduce and even stop concomitant medication with all the advantages of the decrease in drug-related side effects that this can produce. The response to IV lidocaine is not universal. From experience it would seem that about half the fibromyalgia patients who receive IV lidocaine gain relief, although the period of relief can vary from weeks to months. No matter how impressive the relief is, one can expect with certainty that at some stage it will ware off and this can happen suddenly. The infusion can then be repeated as tachyphylaxis does not seem to occur.

Clinical experience would suggest that the magnitude and duration of relief is not dependent on the dose administered, but rather on the speed of infusion. Therefore, in our practice we infuse 1,200 mg of lidocaine over 30h or 12h or 1,000mg over 8h. The 8-h infusion is given as a day case while the 12- and 30-h infusions are administered with a disposable elastomeric infusion device in the patients' home. Side effects with lidocaine infusion are remarkably uncommon with the most frequent being infusion related thrombophlebitis. This can be minimized by placing a segment of a glyceryl trinitrate patch above the infusion site. Our use of IV lidocaine in this fashion and our confidence on it is based on the experience of over 8,000 infusions over the last 10 years.

Lidocaine: topical

Topical lidocaine 5% patches may be used over tender areas. A number of patches can be used simultaneously. A major advantage includes a rapid answer to the question of efficacy, with failure to respond within a day of initiation of treatment being an indication that there is no point in continued therapy.

While the pain of fibromyalgia is widespread, patients often find particular areas more painful than others, and these areas can be targeted with topical agents.

Magnesium

It seems that administration of magnesium can have a marked effect on muscle spasm and muscle-based pain. Unfortunately it is poorly absorbed from the gastrointestinal tract and so for a useful therapeutic effect it needs to be given parenterally. When given by infusion over a number of hours the duration of pain relief can persist for several months. Side effects include postural hypotension and a warm feeling but these both diminish rapidly shortly after the termination of infusion. In our practice we co-administer it with lidocaine to maximize pain relief and reduction in muscle spasm.

Nitrates

The most painful areas in muscles or joints can be targeted with topical nitrates used for their analgesic effect. Clearly, widespread use over many tender areas is inappropriate due to the risk of nitrate headache.

Olanzapine

While use of this atypical neuroleptic agent in patients with fibromyalgia can cause significant pain reduction, many patients discontinue therapy because of weight gain, somnolence, and sedation.

Pramipexole

Pramipexole is a dopamine 3 receptor agonist. Reports are emerging that it can reduce pain, fatigue, and improve overall feeling of well-being in patients with fibromyalgia. Side effects from use include transient anxiety and weight loss.

Quetiapine

While use of this atypical anti-psychotic does not reduce fibromyalgia pain, it can usefully improve overall quality of life scores in patients with this condition.

Tizanadine

This drug is indicated for muscle spasm associated with multiple sclerosis but since it is active on α-adrenoreceptors, it can have analgesic effects as well. It can also cause sedation so can be of use when given at nighttime to aid sleep, relax muscles, and reduce fibromyalgia pain.

Principles of treatment

Fibromyalgia is particularly noted for the lethargy, sleep disturbance, and mood change that accompany pain. While medication can be provided for pain relief, the potential for worsening the accompanying functional impairment that comes with the use of many types of medication may result in those analgesics exacerbating, rather than relieving the patient's overall condition. Therefore, any use of pain-relieving medication should be accompanied by an assessment not only of the pain relief that it produces, but also its overall effect on quality of life. In many cases a modest reduction in pain with no side effects is of more value than substantial pain relief accompanied by undue sedation, weight gain, or cognitive impairment, for example. Further, since patients with fibromyalgia have a variety of other symptoms apart from pain, they may need to take other non-analgesics for these symptoms. Therefore there is a danger that they consume ever increasing numbers of tablets with the consequent dangers in terms of increasing numbers and types of side effects. It is wise, therefore, that when any medication is prescribed, it should be for a defined period of time after which an assessment is undertaken as to its efficacy. Only when that efficacy is proven and the patient is contented that their quality of life is improved by its use should a longer-term prescription be made.

CHAPTER 23

Muscle Spasm and Pain

While the focus of this book is upon pain, muscle spasm is a frequent accompaniment to pain. Indeed, if an abnormal increase in muscle tension persists for any period of time, pain often results while pain of any duration commonly results in muscle spasm. Where muscle spasm and pain are present on their own, treatment can be relatively straightforward. In contrast, where muscle pain results from other conditions, unless that other condition is adequately treated then the response to antispasmodic medication can be disappointing.

When medication that has an effect on muscle spasm and pain is discussed, we refer to the medication as being a muscle relaxant. This should not be confused with the depolarizing and non-depolarizing muscle relaxant classes of medication used in anesthesiological practice which achieves complete relaxation of skeletal muscle to the extent that artificial ventilation of the lungs is required. Those muscle relaxants used in non-anesthesiological practice reduce muscle tone toward that which would be normal without causing paralysis of other muscles.

When muscle spasm occurs, the chronic muscle tension can cause inflammation and pain in the area where that muscle joins onto bone. This area is known as the enthesis and the pain that arises from it as enthetic pain. In time the enthetic pain can feed the muscle spasm to the extent that it, rather than the initial problem that caused the muscle spasm in the first place, causes the muscle spasm to become ongoing. When this enthetic pain occurs, treatment with a muscle relaxant alone is often insufficient. Addition of a non-steroidal anti-inflammatory can reduce the enthetic inflammation while a muscle relaxant reduces muscle tension.

Those drugs which can reduce muscle spasm do so by effects on the central or peripheral nervous system or on the muscle itself. Where the action is on the central nervous system, sedation is a common-side effect. Where the action is on the muscle itself, this adverse effect should be less problematical.

Pain Management: Expanding the Pharmacological Options, Gary J. McCleane. © 2008
Blackwell Publishing, ISBN: 978-1-4051-7823-5.

Clinical presentation of muscle spasm

Muscle spasm presents with a number of features. The patient complains of tightness and stiffness and the location of this is in a non-dermatomal pattern. It can be intermittent, eased by exercise although exacerbations after a period of exercise are common. Where it affects the shoulder girdle and neck, headache is common. Generally heat has a relaxant effect on muscles in spasm, although the duration of relief is very variable. In some situations what is apparent is a mild increase in muscle tone while at the other end of the spectrum there can be complete spasm of the muscle so that it is tightly contracted. Complete spasm of a skeletal muscle can be intermittent and unexpected with sudden onset of incapacitating spasticity.

Along with increases in muscle tone there will often be enthetic pain, that is pain arising from where the muscle joins onto bone. These areas are consistent and so the location of enthetic pain can usefully predict which muscle is in spasm. If it is the paravertebral muscles then pain is felt over the iliac crests and along the 12th rib. If it should be the shoulder girdle muscles then enthetic pain is felt over the base of the skull, mastoid process, suprascapular area, and over the deltoid insertion in the upper arm.

Particular varieties of muscle spasm give rise to identifiable conditions. For example, spasm of the sternomastoid muscle gives rise to torticollis or rye neck where the head is held rotated to the side of the muscle spasm. A further example would be piriformis muscle spasm where pain is felt over the greater trochanter, sciatic notch, and sacral area. This pain is worse on abduction and external rotation of the leg on that side as well as on passage of a bowel motion. Neuropathic pain may also accompany the piriformis muscle spasm as the sciatic nerve is compressed as it passes with the piriformis muscle through the sciatic notch. The tender, tense piriformis muscle can be palpated on digital rectal examination because of the close proximity of the piriformis muscle to the rectum.

Muscle relaxants active on central and peripheral nervous system

Baclofen

Baclofen is the *p*-chlorophenyl derivative of gamma amino butyric acid (GABA). It achieves its effect by being a GABA B agonist and includes among its side effects sedation and confusion. Abrupt cessation of long-term treatment can be associated with a withdrawal reaction. That said, baclofen is usually well tolerated, has a relatively quick onset of action, and is relatively effective in the treatment of muscle spasm. It is also used in the treatment of trigeminal neuralgia.

The exact mechanisms of action of baclofen are not known for certain but seem to involve both pre- and postsynaptic GABA B receptor actions. At the presynaptic site, baclofen decreases calcium conductance with resultant decreased neurotransmitter and excitatory amino acid uptake. At the postsynaptic site, baclofen increases potassium conductance (with resultant neuronal hyperpolarization) and may also inhibit the release of substance P.

Baclofen is available in an oral formulation and also in a form used for intrathecal infusion in patients with refractory spasticity.

Benzodiazepines

Benzodiazepines bind to benzodiazepine receptors located in the terminals of primary fibers leading to increased chloride flux across the terminal membrane with resultant increase in membrane potential.

Side effects of the benzodiazepine group as a whole includes sedation, cognitive impairment, and with prolonged use withdrawal reactions on discontinuation of the drug. Diazepam is frequently used as a muscle relaxant, but if so used its use should be short term and only for acute flare-ups of muscle spasm. Clonazepam appears to possess analgesic and perhaps amnesic properties but has a long half-life so drug accumulation may occur. Lorazepam has some advantage from a pharmacokinetic perspective having a shorter half-life than diazepam or clonazepam and may be used in preference, particularly in the elderly.

Carisoprodol

This agent is primarily metabolized in the liver with multiple metabolites including meprobamate. As metabolism is dependent on deacetylation via the liver micro enzyme CYP 2C19* which a proportion of the population have a deficiency of, there exists "poor metabolizers" of this drug who are at increased risk of experiencing concentration-based side effects such as drowsiness, hypotension, and central nervous system depression at otherwise "normal" doses. There is some risk of respiratory depression with carisoprodol, this risk being increased by the co-administration of propoxyphene.

While the exact mode of action of carisoprodol is not established, it may be that flumazenil may have a role in reversing carisoprodol toxicity.

Cyclobenzaprine

This compound has a tricyclic structure very similar to amitriptyline. Not surprisingly, therefore, it shares a propensity to cause anticholinergic side effects with the Tricyclic Antidepressants (TCAs).

It can be of use in patients with acute and intermittent musculoskeletal conditions including low back pain, muscle spasm, and fibromyalgia.

Local anesthetic nerve blocks

Some nerves have a sensory function, others a motor function, and some subserve both. Where a nerve supplies a motor function alone, blockade of that nerve can cause muscle relaxation in the absence of skin anesthesia. Despite the fact that the deposition of a local anesthetic beside a nerve causes only a short-term blockade of that nerve, prolonged relief of muscle spasm may occur. Often a corticosteroid is added to the local anesthetic in the hope that it will prolong its nerve blocking effect and the corticosteroid may achieve this goal by virtue of its ability to block sodium channels (like the local anesthetic) and if a long-acting corticosteroid is used, then this sodium channel blockade may also be of long duration.

An example of a specific nerve block that can be highly effective in reducing muscle spasm is an accessory nerve block. This nerve supplies the accessory muscle and the anterior portion of the sternomastoid muscle. It has no sensory distribution. It passes close to the skin about one-third of the way down the anterior border of the sternomastoid muscle between the mastoid process and medial end of the clavicle. Deposition of local anesthetic and corticosteroid around the anterior border of the sternomastoid muscle at this location can be a very effective treatment of torticollis. A further example of use of a local anesthetic in the treatment of muscle spasm would be a lumbar epidural injection where the local anesthetic blocks nerves to paravertebral muscles and also to many of the structures which may have initiated the low back pain and caused the muscles to become spasmodic.

Magnesium

Oral administration of magnesium is ineffective because of the poor absorption of the substance from the gut. Therefore it is usually given by the parenteral route. When magnesium is infused over a number of hours, the relief of muscle spasm that can occur can persist for many weeks and even months. Side effects associated with infusion include postural hypotension and a warm feeling felt over the entire body.

Methocarbamol

Methocarbamol is a carbamate derivative of guaifenesin and is structurally related to mephenerin. It is available in both oral and parenteral formulations.

Orphenadrine

Orphenadrine is a monomethylated derivative of diphenhydramine. Centrally acting antihistamines such as this exhibits muscle relaxant and analgesic properties, although the muscle relaxant effect of orphenadrine may also be attributable to its modulating effect of the raphe-spinal serotinergic systems as well.

Orphenadrine also seems to exhibit the characteristics of an *N*-methly-D-aspartate (NMDA) receptor antagonist and this may also account for some of its possible analgesic effects.

Side effects associated with orphenadrine use are partially related to its anticholinergic action and therefore include dry mouth, urinary retention, confusion, blurred vision, agitation, and restlessness.

Orphenadrine is often presented in combination with acetaminophen, aspirin, and non-steroidal anti-inflammatory drugs.

Tizanadine

Tizanadine is an imidazoline derivative that is structurally related to clonidine. Like clonidine, it is an α_2-adrenoreceptor agonist. Its effect, mediated by this receptor, is to cause a direct inhibition of release of excitatory amino acids and a concomitant inhibition of facilitatory coeruleospinal pathways. It is known that epidural and spinal administration of clonidine with local anesthetics opioid combinations is associated with enhanced analgesia and it would therefore be expected that tizanidine may also have analgesic properties.

Somnolence is one of the most frequent side effects of tizanadine use. Its elimination half-life is between 1 and 3 h so it can be administered up to four times daily with a greater proportion of the total daily dose being given at night to augment sleep both because of its hypnotic properties and because muscle relaxation and pain relief may allow a more uninterrupted nights rest.

Muscle relaxants active at nerve endings

Botulinum toxin

Botulinum is a product of the anaerobic bacterium, *Clostridum botulinum*. Of the seven known immunologically distinct serotypes of these extremely potent neurotoxins, types A, B, C1, D, E, F, and G, types A and B are the only types available for routine clinical practice. Two type A preparations, Botox® (Allergan, Inc. Irvine, CA) and Dysport (Ipsen Ltd., Berkshire, UK), have been developed for commercial use and while Dysport is currently being evaluated in the US, only Botox® is available in the US at this time. Type B toxin is currently commercially available as Myobloc™ in the US and as Neurobloc in Europe. While each of these neurotoxins is similar in that they are proteins, they vary with respect to molecular weight, mechanism of action, duration of effect, and adverse effects. The bacteria synthesize each toxin initially as a single chain polypeptide. Bacterial proteases then "nick" both type A as well as type B proteins resulting in a di-chain structure consisting of one heavy and one light chain. Type A is nicked more than Type B and there is less than a 50% homology between the two toxins.

The mechanism of action of these toxins was initially linked to their ability to inhibit the release of acetylcholine from cholinergic nerve terminals; however, for many years it has been generally acknowledged that this effect does not appear to explain the apparent analgesic activity of some of these toxins. In fact much recent research has been directed toward examining other potential and actual mechanisms of action of these toxins that might better explain its analgesic effects. Inhibition of the release of glutamate, substance P, and calcitonin-gene related peptide reduced afferent input to the central nervous system through effects of the toxins on muscle spindles, and other possible effects on pain transmission independent of the effect on cholinergic transmission of these neurotoxins have been proposed based upon the results of many laboratory experiments in which it has been proposed that through a mechanism similar to that which inhibits the release of acetylcholine, these other neurotransmitters are inhibited as well.

The mechanism by which acetylcholine is released by these neurotoxins is a multi-step process. At present, it is clearly much better understood than the mechanism by which these neurotoxins may exert their analgesic effects, although much work has been recently completed regarding its potential analgesic effect. The toxin must be internalized into the synaptic terminal for it to exert its anticholinergic effect. The first step in this process is the binding of the toxin to a receptor on the axon terminals of the cholinergic terminals. Each botulinum toxin serotype binds specifically to its own receptor irreversibly and each neither binds to nor inhibits the other serotypes' receptor. After the toxin is bound, an endosome is formed that carries the toxin into the axon terminal. The final step involves cleavage of one of the known synaptic proteins which are required for acetylcholine to be released by the axon. Botulinum toxins A, E, and C cleave synaptosome-associated protein – 25 (SNAP-25). Botulinum toxins B, D, F, and G cleave synaptobrevin also known as vesicle-associated membrane protein (VAMP). Botulinum toxin type C also cleaves syntaxin. The specific manner in which each toxin type may cleave the synaptic protein as well the specific differences in effect on inhibiting acetylcholine as well as other neurotransmitter release is under active investigation, is quite fascinating but it is beyond the scope of this chapter. In addition, it is not presently known how these differences translate into various observed beneficial as well as adverse effects.

Following injection of the toxin into the muscle, weakness occurs within a few days to a week, peaks most often within 2 weeks, and then gradually resolves with a slow return to baseline. The recovery of strength is associated with sprouting of the affected axon, and the return, for example, of cholinergic synaptic activity to the original nerve terminals. Regeneration of the cleaved synaptic protein is also required for recovery

to occur. The duration of the clinical effect of the currently available neurotoxins appears to be approximately 3 months but may clearly vary from
individual to individual. Additionally, the possible differences in duration
of action of these toxins for different clinical conditions, for example, cervical dystonia vs. migraine headache vs. chronic low back pain has not
been well studied to date. In my clinical experience, the analgesic effect of
botulinum toxin depends upon the serotype used (type A – Botox typically
longer than type B – Myobloc) but is almost always less than 12 weeks.

Perhaps one of the major drawbacks of botulinum toxin use is its cost.
One could therefore argue that before its use is considered a degree of
certainty about the presence of muscle spasm should be present, possibly
accompanied by a response, even if it is partial, to muscle relaxant medication. Further, given that muscle spasm may exist on its own or be precipitated by another condition, such as prolapsed intervertebral disk, facet joint
degeneration or ligament damage, response to botulinum toxin if used on
its own can only be partial if the initiating condition is not adequately dealt
with. If the muscle spasm is present as the only condition, then it is likely
that the response to botulinum toxin may be more complete.

Muscle relaxants active on muscle

Dantrolene

Dantrolene is unusual among the muscle relaxant drugs in that it works
directly on skeletal muscle. It achieves its effect by an action on calcium
uptake by the sarcoplasmic reticulum. Dantrolene is used in the treatment
of malignant hyperpyrexia, a condition occasionally triggered by anesthetic agents and in which intense muscle spasm is a predominant feature.
In those individuals thought to be susceptible to malignant hyperpyrexia,
dantrolene can be used in a prophylactic fashion.

When used in the treatment of muscle spasm and spasticity, a gradual
escalation of dose to an effective level is used. Consequently, dantrolene
is of little use in the immediate treatment of a flare-up of muscle spasm,
but rather has value in the longer-term management of muscle-based
pain. Dantrolene can affect liver function and so periodic blood sampling
to assess liver function should be carried out.

Miscellaneous

A variety of other agents are used by some in the treatment of muscle
spasm and pain. The evidence that supports their use is anecdotal:
• Quinine sulfate (leg cramps)
• Diphenhydramine hydrochloride
• Procainamide

- Phenytoin
- Propoxyphene
- Tricyclic antidepressants
- Cyproheptadine
- Chlorpromazine
- Dronabinol
- L-Threonine (a precursor of glycine)
- Cannabinoids

CHAPTER 24

Tendinopathies

Pain arising from tendons is common and often successfully treated with anti-inflammatories and simple analgesics and recourse to other measures is unnecessary. However, on occasions thought needs to be given to how the more resistant cases of tendonitis can be treated.

Tendon pain is often precipitated either where there is repetitive movement of that tendon or where surrounding structures are abnormal and the movement of the tendon against that structure causes abrasion and consequent inflammation of the tendon. If the tendon normally passes through a restricted area, for example, a bony canal, then inflammation can cause tendon swelling with an increased chance of tendon abrasion in that restricted space. When the tendon becomes inflamed and painful, muscle spasm in the connected muscle often occurs so that pain is experienced not only over the portion of the tendon that is inflamed, but also over the wider area of the supplying muscle. When the patient restricts movement to minimize pain, then the adjacent joint may become stiff and sore. Therefore what starts as a fairly simple disorder may become complicated with pain arising from a variety of adjacent structures. In the longer term, tendon inflammation may lead to calcification and even tendon rupture. Therefore, prompt and efficient treatment can minimize the risk of chronicity and disability.

If one accepts that primary treatment of a tendinitis is with non-steroidal anti-inflammatories (administered topically or orally) and with simple analgesics, then the question arises of what can be tried in the face of failure of these simple remedies. A list of possible alternatives will be presented followed by a suggested treatment algorithm (Figure 24.1).

Topical options

Glyceryl trinitrate

We have seen earlier that the topical application of nitrates in the form of glyceryl trinitrate (GTN) can have both an analgesic and anti-inflammatory

Pain Management: Expanding the Pharmacological Options, Gary J. McCleane. © 2008 Blackwell Publishing, ISBN: 978-1-4051-7823-5.

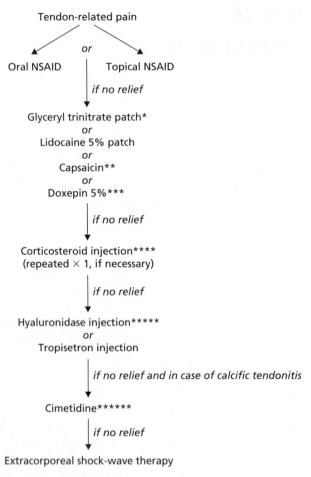

*Glyceryl trinitrate patch, 5 mg per 24 h, 1/4 to 1/2 patch topically daily.
**A 0.025% capsaicin topically four times daily for at least 1 month.
***A 5% doxepin cream topically four times daily for at least 1 month.
****For example, triamcinolone acetonide 20–40 mg with 5–10 ml 0.25% bupivicaine.
*****1,500–3,000 IU Hyaluronidase in 5–10 ml 0.25% bupivicaine.
******200 mg orally twice daily for 3 months.

Figure 24.1 Suggested treatment.

effect and that this effect is achieved by a mechanism distinct and different from that of the NSAIDs. Therefore, as well as being potentially efficacious, it lacks the peptic and other side effects of conventional NSAIDs.

An example of the potential efficacy of GTN in the treatment of the pain of tendinopathy comes from the study of Hunte and Lloyd-Smith (2005). They studied 65 patients whose average duration of pain from their Achilles tendon condition was 16 months, with a range of 4–147 months, emphasizing the potentially chronic nature of this condition. They used a topical patch formulation of GTN which was divided into segments for application over the painful area. When pain and a variety of measures of ankle mobility were considered, those treated with GTN had a greater chance of achieving symptom alleviation than the placebo group. Interestingly, headache, an expected side effect of nitrate use, was reported in 53% of the GTN group, but also by 45% of the placebo group.

Paoloni and colleagues (2004) also studied patients with Achilles tendinopathy. They found that after 6 months of treatment, 78% in the GTN group was asymptomatic as compared to 49% in the placebo group. The fact that after 6 months use patients continued to gain relief suggests that the tachyphylaxis described when nitrates are used to treat angina pectoris may not be encountered when they are used in pain treatment.

The GTN is not only effective in the treatment of Achilles tendon pain. Berrazueta and colleagues (1996) studied 20 patients with supraspinatus tendonitis. The subjects were randomized to receive either a GTN patch (5 mg per 24 h) or a placebo patch. Within 48 h of commencement of treatment, those patients receiving GTN patch treatment recorded a fall of just over 2.5 points on a 10 cm visual analog score of pain. Those in the placebo group recorded no change in pain. Only two patients in the GTN group reported a headache. This study confirms that the pain-relieving effect of topically applied GTN can be rapid and when taken in conjunction with the results of the previously described studies which confirm a long-term effect, it suggests that topical GTN can be a treatment for both the acute and chronic pain associated with tendon pathology.

Lidocaine 5% patch

This lidocaine-containing patch has a verified effect in certain pain conditions and in particular postherpetic neuralgia. While no trial evidence confirms a pain-relieving effect in tendon-related pain, anecdotal evidence, and indeed logic, suggests that it can have such an effect. Only a small amount of the lidocaine contained within the patch is actually released and therefore its effect is local, not systemic. Consequently side effects are relatively uncommon and innocuous. Skin rash and irritation at the application site are perhaps the most frequent complications of use.

Capsaicin

Again capsaicin has a verified effect in a broad range of conditions ranging from neuropathic pains to osteoarthritis, but not specifically tendon-related pain. That said, there is no reason to suggest that it is ineffective in those with tendon-related pain and practical experience confirms this. Capsaicin achieves its effect by reversibly depleting the neurotransmitter substance P and also decreasing the density of epidermal nerve fibers, again in a reversible fashion. Repeated application is required for the effect to be achieved and so a trial of application for up to 1 month is required to gauge success. Burning discomfort at the application site usually decreases with sustained use but can also be reduced by the co-administration of GTN.

Tricyclic antidepressants

Oral tricyclic antidepressants (TCAs) are frequently used in the treatment of chronic pain conditions. However, their use is frequently associated by a variety of side effects including dry mouth, sedation, and weight gain. Recent evidence suggests that TCAs can have a peripheral, as well as central effect, and that this effect is achieved by interaction with peripheral adenosine receptors and sodium channels. Therefore, topical application of a TCA can be used as a method of pain relief, although this pain-relieving effect can take several weeks to become apparent. Side effects with topically applied TCAs are infrequent and non-serious. If over-applied, however, systemic side effects, as seen with oral TCAs, can occur. Currently the TCA doxepin is available in a 5% topically applied formulation.

Muscle relaxants

When tendon inflammation occurs, the attached muscle often becomes spasmodic and painful, compounding the experienced pain. Provision of a simple muscle relaxant drug, such as baclofen, along with specific treatment of the tendinitis, can hasten the cessation of symptoms.

Injections

Steroids

Local injection of corticosteroids is a popular and apparently effective method of treatment for a broad range of painful tendon conditions. Usually this corticosteroid is co-administered with a local anesthetic such as lidocaine or bupivicaine. If a local anesthetic is used, then a fairly rapid reduction in pain confirms that the injection has been placed sufficiently close to the painful area for the corticosteroid to have a chance of alleviating the condition. However, this reduction in pain is often temporary as the effect of the local anesthetic wears off before the corticosteroid has a chance to begin its effect.

While corticosteroid injection is a well-tried method of treatment, a number of side effects can accrue from its use:
- local lipoatrophy producing a depression in the skin at the site of injection
- tendon weakening (especially relevant in weight-bearing tendons such as the Achilles tendon)
- local telangectasia at the injection site
- systemic effects if corticosteroid injection is repeatedly carried out

In terms of the evidence of effect of this form of treatment, an example is given in the meta-analysis of the use of corticosteroid injections for painful shoulders carried out by Arroll and Goodyear-Smith (2005). They found that the "Numbers needed to treat" (NNT), that is, the number of patients needing to receive the treatment for one to gain a 50% reduction in symptoms was 3.3 when this injection was used for rotator cuff tendonitis. The relative risk for improvement when corticosteroid injection was compared to an oral NSAID was 1.43 suggesting that corticosteroid injection (sub-achromial or intra-articular) was, on balance, more effective than an oral NSAID.

So evidence and clinical experience suggest that corticosteroid injection is a potentially effective treatment for tendon-related pain. However, there are many unanswered questions:

- Does the addition of a local anesthetic make any difference to the long-term results of corticosteroid injection?
- Which corticosteroid produces maximum effect (triamcinolone, prednisolone, methylprednisolone, hydrocortisone, depomedrone, or betamethasone)?
- What dose of corticosteroid produces maximum benefit and minimal risk?
- What is a safe dosing interval for corticosteroid injection?

Hyaluronidase

Hyaluronidase is currently most frequently used in conjunction with local anesthetics in peri-bulbar eye blocks where it helps the spread of the local anesthetic. It acts by breaking down soft tissue adhesions and as such can help break down the adhesions that occur with inflammatory conditions of tendons and their sheaths. Injection of Hyaluronidase into a tendon sheath can achieve results comparable with those of corticosteroid injection, but without the potential adverse effects of corticosteroid use. That said, evidence for such an effect is currently lacking.

Tropisetron

Tropisetron belongs to the 5HT$_3$ antagonist group of drugs. This group has been marketed for its antiemetic effect which is most well established in the fields of postoperative nausea and vomiting and in chemotherapy-induced nausea. More recently it has been shown that 5HT$_3$ antagonists, when given systemically, can also have an analgesic effect on the pain associated with fibromyalgia and irritable bowel syndrome and even in patients with neuropathic pain. This effect is produced by their specific action on the NK1-expressing neurones in the superficial laminae of the dorsal horn. These NK1-expressing neurones contain receptors for substance P.

However, Stratz and colleagues (2002) have shown that local, as opposed to systemic, administration of tropisetron can reduce the pain associated with tendinopathies. They compared local injection of tropisetron with an injection of a combination of dexamathasone (10 mg) and lidocaine and assessed pain daily for 7 days and then after 3 months. They found that injection of tropisetron produced the same relief as dexamathasone at all measurement times and that this effect was on rest and movement pain. They speculated that the effect of tropisetron was due to its blocking of $5HT_3$ receptors and an inhibition of substance P release.

 The potential advantage of such use of tropisetron would be that steroid-related side effects could be avoided. There are, however, a number of unanswered questions. Is this effect shared by all $5HT_3$ antagonists? How does the effect of tropisetron compare to other steroids such as triamcinolone or depomedrone? Is there a bell-shaped dose–response curve when tropisetron is used in this fashion as there is when it is used systemically in the treatment of fibromyalgia and is the effect of tropisetron when used to treat the pain associated with a tendinopathy a purely local effect or is there a central effect as well?

Tenoxicam

One would expect that the NSAID tenoxicam, when given systemically, would have the same chance of giving pain relief as any other NSAID. Itzkowitch and colleagues (1996) report that weekly peri-articular injections of tenoxicam (20 mg) gave significant pain relief to patients with painful shoulders, including those with rotator cuff tendinitis when compared to placebo injections. This interesting result leaves a number of questions unanswered. First, is this a local effect or an effect consequent on systemic absorption of tenoxicam? Second, is this effect individual to tenoxicam, or is it shared by other NSAIDs? Still, the fact that weekly injections of this NSAID gave significant relief when the half-life of the drug can be measured in hours, not in days, is intriguing.

Oral options

Cimetidine

It is known that the H_2 antagonist cimetidine decreases calcium levels and can be used with advantage in patients with hyperparathyroidism. When calcium is deposited in the shoulder joint region, impairment of function and pain commonly result. Yokoyama and colleagues (2003) describe 16 patients with chronic calcific tendinitis treated with cimetidine for 3 months. They found that pain scores (100 mm visual analog scale) fell from 63 to 14 mm and that 63% of patients became pain-free. In 56% of their patients, calcium deposits disappeared while in only 25% did they remain unchanged. While this was not a randomized, placebo-controlled trial, the results certainly merit consideration if only because no other pharmacological therapy offers the hope of decalcification of previously calcified tendon.

Others

Nerve blocks

When a noxious event occurs, and particularly when that irritation is prolonged, a number of changes occur that include a "sensitization" of the nerve that travels to that area. Therefore, in the case of tendon pain, while the inflammation is around the tendon and its enveloping structures, the nerve to that region becomes sensitized, excitable, and ultimately contributes to the pain experienced. Therefore, interventions of that nerve can reduce the overall experience of pain. This is best exemplified by suprascapular nerve blocks. Shanahan and colleagues (2003) describe the results of their study on 83 people with shoulder pain who were randomized to receive either a suprascapular nerve block with bupivicaine and methylprednisolone or subcutaneous saline injection. They found that after 1, 4, and 12 weeks the group that received the suprascapular nerve block showed significant improvement in all pain and disability pain scores measured.

Dahan and colleagues (2000) randomized patients to receive thrice weekly suprascapular nerve blocks with either bupivicaine alone or saline as a placebo. Two weeks after the last injection there was a 64% reduction in pain scores in the active treatment group as compared to 13% in the placebo group. What the long-term results were is not clear and therefore the issue of the benefit or lack of benefit of the addition of corticosteroid to the local anesthetic is not addressed.

Extracorporeal shock-wave therapy

A number of studies and case reports have suggested that extracorporeal shock-wave therapy can be useful in the treatment of calcific rotator cuff tendonitis but not in the non-calcific variety. In addition to providing symptom alleviation, a reduction or complete removal of the calcific deposit may occur. For example, Wang and colleagues (2003) found that after treatment with extracorporeal shock-wave therapy in patients with calcific rotator cuff tendonitis, complete dissolution of calcium deposits occurred in 57% with a further 15% of subjects having a partial dissolution. In contrast, in the control group 83% of subjects had no change in their calcium deposits.

Harniman and colleagues (2004) have undertaken a systematic review of the use of extracorporeal shock-wave therapy in patients with calcific and non-calcific tendonitis of the rotator cuff. As is common with such reviews, they found that many studies were weakened by small sample size, randomization issues, blinding and treatment provider bias, and inadequate outcome measures. They concluded that there is moderate evidence that high energy extracorporeal shock-wave therapy is effective in treating chronic calcific rotator cuff tendonitis when the shock waves are focused at the calcific deposit. They also concluded that there is moderate evidence that low energy extracorporeal shock-wave therapy is not effective for treating chronic non-calcific rotator cuff tendonitis, although that conclusion was based on only one high-quality study which was underpowered.

One word of caution is offered by Durst and colleagues (2002) who report a single patient who appeared to develop osteonecrosis of the humeral head after extracorporeal shock-wave therapy.

Hyperbaric oxygen

A single animal study suggests that hyperbaric oxygen may have a beneficial effect on tendinopathy. Hsu and colleagues (2004) induced tendinopathy in rabbits' patellar tendons and treated the animals with hyperbaric oxygen, delivered at 2.5 atmospheres for 120 min on 30 daily sessions or with normobaric room air. After 6 weeks treatment animals were sacrificed and examined histologically. Those treated with hyperbaric oxygen showed cellular changes that indicated healing with greater frequency than animals treated with normobaric room air. They suggested that hyperbaric oxygen may have increased collagen synthesis and collagen cross-link formation during the early healing process.

Perhaps the greatest problem with this form of treatment, if the results can be validated in humans, is the repetitive nature of the treatment with multiple sessions of hyperbaric oxygen being necessary for improvement to occur.

Bibliography

Glyceryl trinitrate

Berrazueta JR, Losada A, Poveda J et al. Successful treatment of shoulder pain syndrome due to supraspinatus tendonitis with transdermal nitroglycerin. A double blind study. *Pain* 1996; 66: 63–7.

Hunte G, Lloyd-Smith R. Topical glyceryl trinitrate for chronic Achilles tendinopathy. *Clin J Sport Med* 2005; 15: 116–17.

Paoloni JA, Appleyard RC, Nelson RC, Murrell GA. Topical nitric oxide application in the treatment of chronic extensor tendinosis at the elbow: a randomized, double-blinded, placebo-controlled clinical trial. *Am J Sports Med* 2003; 31: 915–20.

Paoloni JA, Appleyard RC, Nelson J, Murrell GA. Topical glyceryl trinitrate treatment of chronic noninsertional Achilles tendinopathy. A randomised, double-blind, placebo-controlled trial. *J Bone Joint Surg Am* 2004; 86: 916–22.

Corticosteroids

Arroll B, Goodyear-Smith F. Corticosteroid injections for painful shoulder: a meta-analysis. *Br J Gen Pract* 2005; 55: 224–8.

Tropisetron

Stratz T, Farber L, Muller W. Local treatment of tendinopathies: a comparison between tropisetron and depot corticosteroids combined with local anesthetics. *Scand J Rheumatol* 2002; 31: 366–70.

Stratz T, Varga B, Muller W. Treatment of tendopathies with tropisetron. *Rheumatol Int* 2002; 22: 219–21.

Tenoxicam
Itzkowitch D, Ginsberg F, Leon M et al. Peri-articular injection of tenoxicam for painful shoulders: a double-blind, placebo controlled trial. *Clin Rheumatol* 1996; 15: 604–9.

Cimetidine
Yokoyama M, Aona H, Takeda A, Morita K. Cimetidine for chronic calcifying tendinitis of the shoulder. *Reg Anesth Pain Med* 2003; 28: 248–52.

Nerve blocks
Dahan TH, Fortin L, Pelletier M et al. Double blind randomized clinical trial examining the efficacy of bupivicaine suprascapular nerve blocks in frozen shoulder. *J Rheumatol* 2000; 27: 1464–9.

Shanahan EM, Ahern M, Smith M et al. Suprascapular nerve block (using bupivicaine and methylprednisolone acetate) in chronic shoulder pain. *Ann Rheum Dis* 2003; 62: 400–6.

Extracorporeal shock-wave therapy
Cosentino R, De Stefano R, Selvi E et al. Extracorporeal shock wave therapy for chronic calcific tendinitis of the shoulder: single blind study. *Ann Rheum Dis* 2003; 62: 248–50.

Durst HB, Blatter G, Kuster MS. Osteonecrosis of the humeral head after extracorporeal shock-wave lithotripsy. *J Bone Joint Surg Br* 2002; 84: 744–6.

Gerdesmeyer L, Wagenpfeil S, Haake M et al. Extracorporeal shock wave therapy for the treatment of chronic calcifying tendonitis of the rotator cuff: a randomized controlled trial. *JAMA* 2003; 290: 2573–80.

Harniman E, Carette S, Kennedy C, Beaton D. Extracorporeal shock wave therapy for calcific and noncalcific tendonitis of the rotator cuff: a systematic review. *J Hand Ther* 2004; 17: 132–51.

Peters J, Luboldt W, Schwarz W et al. Extracorporeal shock wave therapy in calcific tendinitis of the shoulder. *Skeletal Radiol* 2004; 33: 712–18.

Perlick L, Luring C, Bathis H et al. Efficacy of extracorporeal shock-wave treatment for calcific tendinitis of the shoulder: experimental and clinical results. *J Orthop Sci* 2003; 8: 777–83.

Speed CA, Richards C, Nichols D et al. Extracorporeal shock-wave therapy for tendonitis of the rotator cuff. A double-blind, randomised, controlled trial. *J Bone Joint Surg Br* 2002; 84: 509–12.

Wang CJ, Yang KD, Wang FS et al. Shock wave therapy for calcific tendonitis of the shoulder: a prospective clinical study with two-year follow-up. *Am J Sports Med* 2003; 31: 425–30.

Hyperbaric oxygen
Hsu RW, Hsu WH, Tai CL, Lee KF. Effect of hyperbaric oxygen therapy on patellar tendinopathy in a rat model. *J Trauma* 2004; 57: 1060–4.

CHAPTER 25
Low Back Pain

Few areas of pain control are more difficult than the management of low back pain. While the majority of sufferers can expect a rapid resolution of symptoms with active mobilization and then passage of time, others progress to having a chronic disabling condition for which there is little uniformity in treatment. At the early stages provision of simple analgesics and anti-inflammatories may allow mobilization, at later stages these types of medication may contribute little to treatment.

Low back pain is undoubtedly a complex condition, both in terms of the genesis of the pain and in the interpretation of the pain by the treating physician. A variety of schools of thought govern treatment with at one end of the spectrum some having the opinion that the medics have little or no part in the treatment of chronic low back pain to those who take a highly interventional approach. It is necessary to have a methodology for the interpretation of the symptoms and signs that occur for a suggested treatment regimen to be put in place. Given the diversity of opinion that surrounds the treatment of low back pain, such a methodology is likely to be somewhat controversial and not accepted by all. In this chapter an opinion on the diagnosis of low back pain will be given followed by suggested treatments for the individual component pains found in those with low back pain.

Diagnosis

It is suggested that the term "low back pain" merely describes the occurrence of pain in a particular location and is not a diagnosis any more than *leg pain* or *head pain* would be a diagnosis either. Low back pain occurs because of injury or irritation to those structures that are found in the back. In some cases single structures are affected, while in others multiples of structures give rise to pain. Each individual structure can give rise to specific and diagnostic symptoms and signs that are individually and

Pain Management: Expanding the Pharmacological Options, Gary J. McCleane. © 2008 Blackwell Publishing, ISBN: 978-1-4051-7823-5.

specifically treatable. Therefore, pain can arise, in general, from the following structures:

- muscle
- enthesis
- ligament
  - interspinous
  - sacroiliac
  - sacrococcygeal
- joint
  - facet
  - sacroiliac
  - sacrococcygeal
- nerve
- bone
  - vertebra
  - coccyx

An aid to diagnosis is the presence of referred or radiated pain. This can give insight into the location of the causative injury and to possible causes of the injury. Both are felt in a dermatomal distribution corresponding to the dermatomal level at which the injury occurs. Referred pain is experienced as a toothache like constant pain, while radiated pain has neuropathic features and can include paresthesia, burning, allodynia, lancinating pain, and numbness. When the source of the pain is to one side of the midline, then the consequent referred or radiated pain is to the appropriate dermatome on that side. Where it is from a midline structure, then the referred pain is often felt bilaterally.

An aide memoir to diagnosis is contained in Table 25.1.

Treatment

All treatment comes with the proviso that active mobilization is an essential facet of treatment. In some individuals a single cause of back pain can be identified, while in others several structures generate pain and specific treatment of each will be required to increase the chance of therapeutic success. In still further cases, when an individual type of pain originating from a single structure is identified and treated, further sources of pain become obvious either because they were masked by the original pain or because stress is put on these other structures during mobilization and so a process of intermittent re-evaluation and adjustment of treatment is often required.

For the sake of simplicity, treatments for pain from individual structures will be separately considered (Table 25.2).

Table 25.1 Aides to the diagnosis of back pain.

Structure giving rise to pain	Location of pain	Type of pain	Referred pain	Radiated pain	Associated factors
Muscle, paravertebral	Paravertebral region	Tightness Spasmodic Stiffness			Eased by heat Postexercise exacerbation Worse on lateral flexion Associated with muscle tension headache
Muscle, piriformis	Sciatic area over greater trochanter	Tightness			Worse on bowel movement and abduction/external rotation of leg Tenderness over sciatic notch Palpable spasm of piriformis muscle on rectal examination
Enthetic pain	Over enthetic areas				May be palpable muscle spasm
Ligament: interspinous	Midline	Localized Sharp	May be referred bilaterally		Worse on spine flexion Tenderness between spinous processes
Ligament: sacroiliac	Over sacroiliac area	Localized	Referred to back of thigh		Worse on all movements Often associated with palpable thickening of ligament

Ligament: sacrococcygeal	Between coccyx and ischium	Localized	Referred to back of thigh	Localized tenderness to either side of midline in coccygeal area
Joint: facet	Just lateral to midline	Localized	Referred pain to corresponding dermatome	Pain worse on back extension Associated muscle spasm
Joint: sacroiliac	Over sacroiliac area	Localized		Joint tenderness Worse on springing pelvis
Joint: sacrococcygeal	Over sacrococcygeal joint	Localized		Joint tenderness Worse on pressing coccyx
Nerve	Over affected dermatome	Allodynia Paresthesia Lancinating pain Numbness	Affected dermatome	Worse on back flexion May be motor weakness May be abnormal reflexes
Bone: vertebra	Over affected vertebra	Midline pain Localized tenderness	Referred bilaterally	May be associated with neuropathic, ligament, joint, and muscle pain May be history of trauma or osteoporosis
Bone: coccyx	Pain over coccyx	Localized Midline	Referred bilaterally to front of thighs	Worse on coccygeal pressure

Table 25.2 Treatments for pain.

Muscle pain/spasm

Options:
- Muscle relaxant drugs (e.g., baclofen, dantrolene)
- Glyceryl trinitrate patches
- Lidocaine 5% patches
- Topical doxepin
- Intravenous lidocaine
- Epidural clonidine
- L-Carnitine if muscle spasm is long-standing
- Botulinum toxin injection

Enthetic pain

Options:
- Glyceryl trinitrate patches
- Lidocaine 5% patch
- Topical doxepin
- Topical capsaicin
- Injection with corticosteroid or 5HT$_3$ antagonist
- Intravenous lidocaine

Since enthetic pain and muscle spasm usually co-exist, addition of a muscle relaxant can aid the above options in the case of enthetic pain, while reduction of enthetic pain can reduce the tendency for muscle spasm to become self-sustaining.

Ligament pain

Interspinous

Options:
- Glyceryl trinitrate patch
- Lidocaine 5% patch
- Topical capsaicin
- Topical doxepin
- Injection of ligament with corticosteroid or 5HT$_3$ antagonist
- Intravenous lidocaine

Sacroiliac

Options:
- Glyceryl trinitrate patch
- Lidocaine 5% patch
- Topical capsaicin
- Topical doxepin
- Injection of ligament with corticosteroid, hyaluronidase, or 5HT$_3$ antagonist
- Intravenous lidocaine

Sacrococcygeal

Options:
- Glyceryl trinitrate patch
- Lidocaine 5% patch
- Topical capsaicin
- Topical doxepin
- Injection of ligament with corticosteroid or 5HT$_3$ antagonist
- Intravenous lidocaine

Joint

Facet

Options:
- Glyceryl trinitrate patch
- Lidocaine 5% patch

Table 25.2 (Continued)

	– Topical capsaicin	
	– Topical doxepin	
	– Glucosamine	
	– Injection of joint or supplying nerves with corticosteroid or 5HT$_3$ antagonist	
	– Intravenous lidocaine	
	– Epidural corticosteroid injection	
	– Anti-epileptic drug (e.g., lamotrigine) for referred pain	
Sacroiliac Options:	– Glyceryl trinitrate patch	
	– Lidocaine 5% patch	
	– Topical capsaicin	
	– Topical doxepin	
	– Glucosamine	
	– Injection of joint with corticosteroid or 5HT$_3$ antagonist	
	– Intravenous lidocaine	
Sacrococcygeal Options:	– Glyceryl trinitrate patch	
	– Lidocaine 5% patch	
	– Topical capsaicin	
	– Topical doxepin	
	– Injection of joint with corticosteroid or 5HT3 antagonist	
	– Intravenous lidocaine	
Nerve Options:	– Lidocaine 5% patch	*If area of pain is relatively small*
	– Topical capsaicin	
	– Topical doxepin	
	– L-Carnitine	
	– Anti-epileptic drug (e.g., lamotrigine)	
	– Antidepressant (e.g., duloxetine)	
	– Epidural injection with corticosteroid or clonidine	
	– Epidural injection with hyaluronidase in case of postlaminectomy fibrosis	
	– Intravenous lidocaine	
Bone *Vertebra* Options:	– Glyceryl trinitrate patch	
	– Lidocaine 5% patch	*For localized midline pain*
	– Topical capsaicin	
	– Topical doxepin	
	– Glucosamine	*For associated facet joint pain*
	– Facet joint injection with corticosteroid or 5HT$_3$ antagonist	
	– Injection with corticosteroid or 5HT$_3$ antagonist if there is ligament pain	
	– Anti-epileptic drug (e.g., lamotrigine) for associated radiated or referred pain	

(Continued)

Table 25.2 (Continued)

	– Intravenous lidocaine
	– Epidural corticosteroid, clonidine, or hyaluronidase injection
Coccyx	
Options:	– Glyceryl trinitrate patch
	– Lidocaine 5% patch
	– Topical capsaicin
	– Topical doxepin
	– Injection with corticosteroid or $5HT_3$ antagonist
	– Intravenous lidocaine
	– Epidural clonidine injection

CHAPTER 26

Cancer Pain

The philosophy of timely, graded, and appropriate treatment of pain associated with terminal illness is now well established in practice. Significant
advances have been made in both the application of this philosophy and
the availability of drugs that can provide good quality pain relief in the
last few years. There are circumstances, however, where a simpler, and
perhaps unconventional, therapeutic approach to the presenting pain may
provide the same or even superior analgesia, but with less complication by
troubling side effects.

When considering a patient with pain associated with a terminal illness
then in general the pain may be present for the following reasons:
- Because of infiltration or irritation by the tumor into body structures
  (e.g., nerve, viscus, muscle, and bone).
- As a side effect of the treatment provided for the illness (e.g., chemotherapy, radiotherapy, and surgery).
- Due to the terminal illness exacerbating a pre-existing pain condition
  (e.g., immobility exacerbating low back pain).
- May be totally unrelated to the illness (e.g., prolapsed intervertebral
  disk, painful diabetic neuropathy, and osteoarthritis).

There is no unique treatment for *cancer pain* any more than there is for
low back pain or *postoperative pain*. What there is, however, are treatments
verified by clinical trials and extensive practical use. Therefore, opioids are
extensively utilized and most useful. That does not mean to say that they
are the only, and certainly not the optimal, treatment for specific types of
pain. If in the treatment of pain associated with chronic benign disease,
the first step in treatment of, for example a neuropathic pain, is an anti-
epileptic drug, why should it be different in a patient with a life-limiting
condition?

It is suggested, therefore, that in the overall treatment of pain associated
with terminal illness that a diagnosis of which structure is irritated or
traumatized, and hence producing pain, should be made to guide treatment

Pain Management: Expanding the Pharmacological Options, Gary J. McCleane. © 2008
Blackwell Publishing, ISBN: 978-1-4051-7823-5.

using medications known to be most effective and most easily tolerated by the patient for that particular type of pain. Therefore, pharmacological treatment of pain produced by malignant infiltration of a nerve could include topical lidocaine patches, capsaicin, doxepin, oral anti-epileptics, antidepressants, and so on. After all, whether in this example a nerve is injured by tumor, infection, surgical trauma, or metabolic disease, the resultant pain has a uniformity in both the nature and quality of pain produced and consequently in treatment.

It would seem unnecessary therefore to repeat all treatments outlined in previous chapters for pain arising from various body structures. What will now be discussed are some novel options which are more unique to the pain treatment of the terminally ill patient.

Pancreatic pain

The pain associated with pancreatic cancer can be excruciating and difficult to control. When conventional analgesic therapy fails to control pain then consideration may be given to celiac plexus block where a neurolytic solution is placed in this structure with the intention of destroying the sympathetic fibers, which innervate the pancreas and modulate this pain.

An alternative is the use of the adrenoreceptor antagonist phentolamine. This agent is available only in a parenteral formulation. It has shown to be of some value in treating a variety of pain conditions including the visceral pain associated with porphyria, chronic pancreatitis, and complex regional pain syndrome type 1. What unifies these conditions is that at least part of the pain is sympathetically mediated. Given that celiac plexus block destroys sympathetic nerves and reduces pancreatic cancer pain then one would expect phentolamine to temporarily replicate this effect, which it can do. Intravenous infusion given over a 1-day period can reduce pancreatic cancer pain for several weeks at a time. Complications associated with use include palpitations and postural hypotension, which can be minimized if the patient receives a fluid preload prior to commencement of infusion. Unfortunately since nausea and vomiting along with anorexia often complicate pancreatic cancer, the chances of the patient being dehydrated prior to treatment are increased with a commensurate increased chance of palpitations and postural hypotension being produced. The other major side effect is thrombophlebitis at the infusion site, which can be minimized if the phentolamine is well diluted, given into a large vein and if a glyceryl trinitrate patch is placed above the infusion site.

The other potentially valuable treatment is the use of a cholecystokinin antagonist such as proglumide. The partial resistance of pancreatic pain to opioids may be partially due to the fact that the pancreas is sympathetically innervated and also because this gland releases cholecystokinin when damaged with this peptide having an anti-opioid effect. When proglumide is given by infusion over a number of hours, then weeks of relief may be produced. Side effects with this treatment are uncommon. When the patient is taking strong opioids for their pain, the dose can be automatically reduced by about one-third when proglumide is administered. Unfortunately, at present, proglumide is not commercially available.

Other options for the control of pancreatic cancer pain include intravenous (IV) lidocaine and 5HT$_3$ antagonists.

Vertebral fracture pain

Vertebral fracture can result from trauma and is more likely if the vertebral bone is abnormally soft either because of osteoporosis or malignant infiltration. In general the resultant pain is similar whether it is produced by a malignant or non-malignant process. Where vertebral infiltration by tumor occurs, radiotherapeutical treatment is often of benefit. The treatment outlined here is only of the pharmacological variety.

While most fractures result in bone fracture pain, that arising from a vertebral collapse fracture manifests itself according to which vertebral structure, or structures, are irritated by the process itself and also the changes in vertebral architecture that result from the change in bone shape. Consequently, the following structures can give rise to pain, with each possible cause having specific treatments which may help:
• Vertebral body
• Interspinous ligament
• Spinal nerve
• Facet joints
• Paravertebral muscles
• Intervertebral disk
• Spinal cord

Therefore, when assessment is made of a patient with a vertebral collapse fracture, it is important to determine which combination of structures are giving rise to pain. Where there are neuropathic elements, such as paresthesia, lancinating pain, allodynia, and numbness, one can suspect either spinal cord or spinal nerve root irritation. Where the symptoms are bilateral and associated with muscle weakness and affect the patient below a certain level, then it is likely that spinal cord irritation is occurring. If the symptoms are radicular and unilateral, then there is a greater chance that they arise from spinal nerve root compromise. The resultant neuropathic pain can be treated as outlined in earlier chapters.

When there is localized tenderness in the back, then localized treatment has some chance of helping. The treatment of pain arising from anterior longitudinal ligament and parts of the intervertebral disks are more problematical as these structures are sympathetically innervated.

Treatments

Interspinous ligament

    Glyceryl trinitrate patch

    Lidocaine 5% patch

    Topical capsaicin

    Topical doxepin

    Injection into the ligament of corticosteroid or $5HT_3$ antagonist

    Intravenous lidocaine

Muscle

    Muscle relaxant (e.g., baclofen, dantrolene)

    Topical doxepin

    Glyceryl trinitrate patch

    Lidocaine 5% patch

    Botulinum toxin

    Intravenous lidocaine

Spinal nerve and spinal cord

    Anti-epileptic drug (e.g., lamotrigine)

    Antidepressant (e.g., duloxetine)

    Intravenous lidocaine

    L-carnitine

    Epidural clonidine

Facet joint

    Glyceryl trinitrate patch

    Lidocaine 5% patch

    Facet joint injection with corticosteroid or $5HT_3$ antagonist

    Intravenous lidocaine

    Anti-epileptic drug for referred pain (e.g., lamotrigine)

    Epidural corticosteroid injection

Vertebral body collapse may cause pain of its own for a relatively short time after fracture. Thereafter the pain usually results from irritation of one of the structures mentioned above. Similarly, prolapsed intervertebral disks usually give rise to pain when they impinge on a spinal nerve or spinal cord so treatment is that of the pain resulting from neural compression.

Visceral pain

Lesions involving a hollow viscus are not a major inducer of pain but should that lesion cause distension of the viscus then pain will result. Given that gut is sympathetically innervated, the resultant pain will have a generalized nature. Conventional pain therapy with opioids can help, but where these opioids impede colonic transit, then further distension may occur.

Pain relief for visceral pain falls into two categories. First, there is general analgesic treatment and second, pharmacological interventions that reduce pain by reducing the causative distension. Considering the latter first, distension can be reduced by administration of corticosteroids, which reduce inflammation around any obstructive stricture, thereby increasing, albeit temporarily, the caliber of the viscus at that point. A further approach is the administration of the like of octreotide which reduces intra-luminal secretion and therefore viscal distension.

There are also a few options for analgesic therapy. Intravenous lidocaine can reduce visceral pain with the duration of relief extending beyond both the period of infusion and the half-life of the drug. $5HT_3$ antagonists can also be of value with the dual benefits of an antiemetic effect along with a possible visceral analgesic effect. A third option is the IV infusion of phentolamine, as outline for the treatment of pancreatic carcinoma-related pain. Again the period of relief produced can extend beyond the duration of infusion and the half-life of this drug.

Chemotherapy-associated pain

Two relatively common consequences of cancer chemotherapy are neuropathy with accompanying neuropathic pain and mucositis.

Chemotherapy-induced neuropathic pain

While this type of neuropathic pain can respond in the same way to treatment as any other type of neuropathic pain, the patient has the twin burdens of the cancer illness and disability produced as a temporary side effect of chemotherapy to endure, and so the imposition of neuropathic pain treatment related side effects needs to be avoided if at all possible. Therefore, the simpler the treatment the better. Particular treatments stand out in this respect. The dietary supplement L-carnitine has the advantages of a low risk of producing side effects and a relatively high chance of helping. Time to effect is also sort. Anecdotal evidence would also suggest that IV lidocaine and oral lamotrigine can both be efficacious and relatively well tolerated by the patient.

Chemotherapy-induced mucositis

When severe, this can severely restrict the patients' desire and ability to take both food and fluids by mouth at the very time when both are so essential. Three unconventional treatments for this condition exist.

1 Oral rinse with doxepin hydrochloride. Among the first reports of a local, peripheral analgesic effect of the tricyclic antidepressants was with oral doxepin rinse with cancer chemotherapy related mucositis. The pain relief produced may be due to the actions of tricyclic antidepressants on sodium channels, opioid, and adenosine receptors, all of which are found peripherally. Despite its sodium channel blocking effect, this is not sufficient to compromise the protective glottic reflexes.

2 Oral rinse with strong opioids such as morphine or fentanyl. Again the effect is probably peripheral and local to the mouth and is achieved because of the presence of peripheral opioid receptors.

3 Oral rinse with cocaine. This has fairly intense local anesthetic effects.

In practice, any one, or combination, of these treatments can be given and can be presented in the form of a lollipop along with a flavoring agent such as orange. These constituents can be frozen so that the patient can also benefit from the coldness of the lollipop which they are sucking.

Pain associated with epidural metastasis

The epidural veins form a portal circulation, which connects the pelvic spinal canal and brain. Through these veins tumor deposit can circulate from pelvic organs, for example, to the brain. When malignant deposits traverse these veins, then tumor can form in the epidural space. Symptoms produced include radicular pain in the dermatome supplied by the spinal nerves at the level of deposit, with this pain being exacerbated by lying flat and exercise. In addition, weakness in muscles supplied by involved spinal nerves is often exacerbated by exercise. Even strong opioids and anti-epileptic drugs are relatively ineffective for this condition. Corticosteroids, on the other hand, can be highly effective in reducing epidural space tumor bulk, with a consequent reduction of the pressure effects of the malignant deposit and hence pain. Steroids can be most effectively administered via epidural injection, although attempts to insert an epidural needle at the level of tumor deposit are inadvisable as the epidural space, normally a potential, rather than actual space, may be full of tumor deposit so a land mark for space location may be lost and so the risk of dural puncture is increased. A safer approach is to insert the epidural needle somewhat distant to the site and feed an epidural catheter toward the level of tumor. Ideally a longer acting, depot steroid preparation, such as triamcinolone, can be used for extended relief. Inevitably, tumor bulk will increase again, but the temporary relief caused by epidural steroid injection can be profound and most useful.

Phantom pain

While one instinctively thinks of phantom limb pain when phantom pain is considered, it may also complicate many surgical procedures that involve amputation. Consequently, patients may experience phantom breast pain after mastectomy or tenesmus after rectal excision. Even more prevalent than phantom pain is phantom awareness, that is the sensation that the amputated appendage is still in place, when, in fact, it has been surgically removed. In the case of tenesmus after rectal excision, care needs to be taken as the onset of tenesmus may represent tumor recurrence as well as a form of phantom pain.

Anecdotal evidence would suggest that the anti-epileptic drugs can be useful in the management of phantom pain, while epidural clonidine can also be of benefit. Intravenous lidocaine can suppress symptoms, but will inevitably need to be repeated as the duration of relief is finite. Added to pharmacological therapy there is the imperative that adequate explanation is given to the patient, as onset of this symptom can be mystifying to the patient.

Suggested Doses and Modes of Administration of Novel Pharmacological Options

Drug	Formulation	Unit dose	Dose escalation	Time to effect	Predominant side effects
Topical					
Glyceryl trinitrate	Patch	$5\,mg\,24\,h^{-1}$	1/4 patch increasing by 1/4 patch daily to 1 patch daily	24 h	Headache Light-headedness Skin rash under patch
Lidocaine	5% patch	1–3 patches daily		24 h	Skin rash at application site
Doxepin	5% cream	Pea-sized application		1–3 weeks	Side effects of oral Tricyclic antidepressant if over applied
Capsaicin	0.025% and 0.075% cream	Pea-sized application		1–4 weeks	Burning/tingling Sneezing
Oral					
L-carnitine	Tablet	500 mg twice daily		2 weeks	Can have antidepressant effect and cause weight loss

Drug	Formulation	Dose	Regimen	Duration	Side effects
Lamotrigine	Tablet	50 mg	50 mg daily increasing by 50 mg weekly to 300 mg Daily (single or divided doses)	6 weeks	Skin rash Lymphadenopathy Insomnia Mastalgia
Ondansetron	Tablet	4 mg	4 mg three times daily	24 h	Headache Constipation
Granisetron	Tablet	2 mg	Once daily	24 h	Headache Constipation
Glucosamine	Tablet	1,500 mg	Once daily	Up to 6 months	
Proglumide	Tablet	200 mg	200 mg twice daily	24 h	Bitter taste of tablet Occasional skin rash
Cimetidine	Tablet	200 mg	200 mg twice daily	2 months	
Clonazepam	Tablet	0.5 mg	1.0–1.5 mg at night	Hours	
Baclofen	Tablet	10 mg	10 mg three times daily	Hours	Nausea Occasional sedation
Dantrolene	Capsule	25 mg	25 mg daily increasing by 25 mg weekly to 100 mg a day	1 month	Nausea Sedation
Intravenous					
Lidocaine	Infusate	1,200 mg	over 30 h	Up to 1 week	Light-headedness Peri-oral tingling Nausea
Lidocaine	Infusate	1,000 mg	over 8 h	Up to 1 week	Light-headedness Peri-oral tingling Nausea
Fosphenytoin	Infusate (IV)	1,500 PE units	Over 24 h	2 days	Light-headedness Nausea

(Continued)

(Continued)

Drug	Formulation	Unit dose	Dose escalation	Time to effect	Predominant side effects
Fosphenytoin	Injectate (IM)	500 PE units	Single dose	hours	Perineal burning sensation
Ondansetron	Injectate	8 mg	Single dose IV or IM	Hours	Pain at injection site Perineal burning Sensation
Granisetron	Injectate	2 mg	Single dose IV or IM	Hours	Headache
Proglumide	Injectate	400 mg	1,200 mg IV over 24 h	24 h	Headache
Adenosine	Injectate		$50\,mcg\,Kg^{-1}\,min^{-1}$ over 60 min	Days	
Infiltration/nerve block/epidural					
Ondansetron	Injectate	8 mg	Single injection	48 h	Headache
Granisetron	Injectate	2 mg	Single injection	48 h	Headache
Clonidine	Injectate	150 mcg	Single epidural injection	48 h	Hypotension Sedation Dry mouth
Hyaluronidase	powder	1,500 IU	3,000 IU dissolved in local anesthetic solution	48 h	
Botulinum A toxin	Powder	100 IU	Multiple injections around site of muscle spasm	1 week	Muscle spasm after injection

Index